Sigmundoscopy
Medical-Psychiatric Consultation-Liaison
The Bases

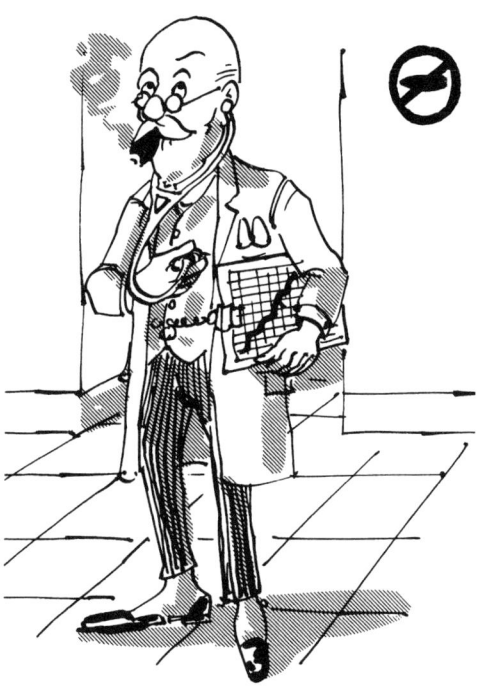

David J. Robinson, M.D., F.R.C.P.C.
Diplomate of the American Board of
Psychiatry & Neurology

Consultation-Liaison Psychiatrist
St. Joseph's Health Center, London, Canada

Rapid Psychler Press

Suite 374
3560 Pine Grove Ave.
Port Huron, Michigan
USA 48060

Suite 263
2-1200 London Rd.
Sarnia, Ontario
Canada N7S 1P4

Toll Free Phone   888-PSY-CHLE (888-779-2453)
Toll Free Fax   888-PSY-CHLR (888-779-2457)
Outside the U.S. & Canada — Phone 519-383-7400
Outside the U.S. & Canada — Fax 519-383-7600
website   www.psychler.com
email   rapid@psychler.com

ISBN 0-9680324-5-1
Printed in the United States of America
©1999, Rapid Psychler Press
First Edition, First Printing

All rights reserved. This book is protected by copyright. No part of this book may be reproduced in any form or by any means without written permission. Unauthorized copying is prohibited by law and will be dealt with by a punitive superego as well as all available legal means (including a lawyer with a Cluster B Personality Disorder).

Please support creativity by not photocopying this book.

All caricatures are purely fictitious. Any resemblance to real people, either living or deceased, is entirely coincidental (and unfortunate). The author assumes no responsibility for the consequences of diagnoses made, or treatment instituted as a result of the contents of this book. These determinations should be made by qualified mental health professionals. Every effort was made to ensure the information in this book was accurate at the time of publication. However, due to the changing nature of the field of psychiatry, the reader is encouraged to consult additional and more recent sources of information.

Dedication

This book is dedicated to those people who helped me on my journey.

- Ali D. Aziz, M.D.
- Peter V. Clarke, M.D.
- Joel Fish, M.D.
- Barry A. Roth, M.D.
- Robert Silver, M.D.

Special Contributors

- Paul I. Steinberg, M.D., F.R.C.P.C.
- Sandra Northcott, M.D., F.R.C.P.C.

Rapid Psychler Press

produces books and presentation media that are:

- comprehensively researched
- well organized
- formatted for ease of use
- reasonably priced
- clinically oriented, and
- include humor that enhances education, and that neither demeans patients nor the efforts of those who treat them

Table of Contents

Author's Foreword	vi-vii
Acknowledgments	viii-ix
Publication Notes	x

Chapter 1
    History & Organization of
    C-L Psychiatry   3

Chapter 2
    Use & Usefulness of
    C-L Psychiatry   55

Chapter 3
    Conducting the Consult   75

Chapter 4
    The Consultation Report   109

Chapter 5
    Implementing the
    Treatment Plan   145

Chapter 6
    Legal & Ethical Aspects   171

The Consultation Process   178
Index   180

Author's Foreword

Two factors which contribute greatly to the stress of medical education are information overload and the often less than helpful teaching approaches of some clinical supervisors.

Prior to entering medical school, most students are enrolled in programs with relatively circumscribed curricula and defined expectations for examinations. Once medical studies have begun, there is an explosion of material which must be learned, and learned well. There has been relatively little attention paid to assist with the daunting task of amalgamating thousands of what at times appear to be unconnected facts. I have rarely heard instructors say to students something along the lines of *"that's more than you need to know about this topic."*

Because clinical skills cannot be learned entirely from textbooks, medical education involves a long apprenticeship. We all depend on experienced teachers to show us how and why things are done a certain way. Unfortunately, this phase of training is frequently seen as a "rite of passage" or "trial by fire." Trainees are often spared little when it comes to difficult or embarrassing situations. A common mindset is that students and residents must prove themselves by traversing (with as little assistance as possible) the same obstacles that faced their supervisors. This sentiment has been aptly referred to as "The Days of the Giants." Supervisors, reminiscing about their difficult days as trainees, often lament that things are much too easy nowadays. Some feel that lending more than cursory assistance to students deprives them of valuable learning opportunities. Inherent in this attitude is that experiencing hardship is the primary factor in building character, and that embarrassment or humiliation are valuable allies in education.

This book is an attempt to help with both information overload and to provide practical recommendations based on many years of clinical work. My primary aim in education and publishing is to

Sigmundoscopy — The Bases

assist others in learning the material as quickly, easily and enjoyably as possible. In order to accomplish this, I develop mnemonics, invent clinical vignettes and rigorously edit the manuscript so that the content is presented as crisply as possible.

The other aspect which sets my books apart from most others is the inclusion of caricatures and other humorous material. I think that if the practitioners of any specialty should have a sense of humor about their work, it would be psychiatrists. While many mental health professionals endorse the use of humor (e.g. in lectures), very few include it in their published work. This book contains humorous illustrations and vignettes which were designed to enhance the educational aspects being presented, not detract from them. I have found humor to be an extremely effective way of adding perspective and keeping interest, which is why it is included here.

Consultation-Liaison (C-L), to me, is the pinnacle of psychiatry. No other area draws upon so many facets of the specialty. This work keeps us in touch both with our medical/surgical colleagues and the years we spent learning about physical illnesses. A well-conducted consult benefits the patient, the patient's family, consultee and trainees, and enhances the reputation of the specialty.

Sigmundoscopy — The Bases was written to provide readers with background information on many aspects of C-L psychiatry, as well as an indepth review of the consultation process. As always, I am interested in feedback and suggestions for future editions.

Keep Psychling!

Dave Robinson

June, 1999
London, Canada

Rapid Psychler Staff

I am very grateful to have the time and talents of these people available to me. Their continual support and enthusiasm were of crucial assistance in the preparation of this text.

- ◆ Brian & Fanny Chapman
- ◆ Monty & Lil Robinson
- ◆ Lisa & Cathy Burgard
- ◆ Nicole & Mark Kennedy
- ◆ Brad Groshok
- ◆ Sam Wilson
- ◆ Dean Avola
- ◆ Dr. Donna Robinson & Dr. Robert Bauer

Acknowledgments

I am indebted to the following people for their support while writing this text and for their assistance in furthering my academic interests:

- Tom Norry, B.Sc.N.
- Sandra Northcott, M.D.
- Lisa Bogue, M.D.
- Thomas Gantert, B.Sc.N.
- Paul Steinberg, M.D.
- Lisa Burgard
- Cathy Burgard
- John Mount, M.D.
- John Craven, M.D.
- Harold Merskey, D.M.

Publication Notes

Terminology
Throughout this book, the term "patient" is used to refer to people who are suffering and seek help. The term is further used to describe those who bear pain without complaint or anger.

The terms "consumer" or "consumer-survivor" reflect an unfortunate trend that is pejorative towards mental health care, labeling it as if it were a trade or business instead of a profession. These terms are also ambiguous, as it is not clear what is being "consumed" or "survived."

Graphics
All of the illustrations in this book are original works of art commissioned by Rapid Psychler Press and are a signature feature of our publications.

Rapid Psychler Press makes available an entire library of color illustrations (including those from this book) as 35mm slides and overhead transparencies. These images are available for viewing and can be purchased from our website — **www.psychler.com**

These images from our color library may be used for presentations.

We request that you respect our copyright and do not reproduce these images in any form for any purpose at any time.

Bolded Terms
Throughout this book, various terms appear in bolded text, which allows for ease of identification. Most of these terms are defined in this text. Some, however, are only mentioned because a detailed description is beyond the scope of this book. Fuller explanations of all of the bolded terms can be found in standard reference texts.

Let's Go!

Sigmundoscopy
Medical-Psychiatric Consultation-Liaison The Bases

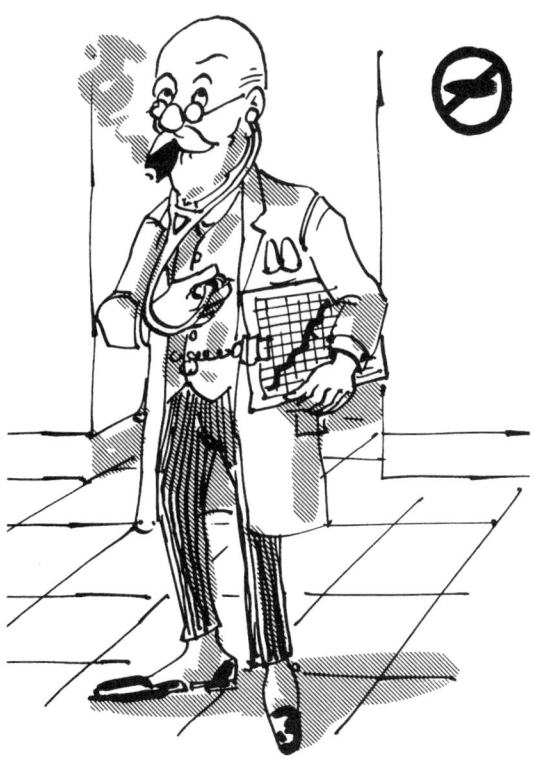

"In order to cure the human body, it is necessary to have knowledge of the whole of things."

Hippocrates

Sigmundoscopy — The Bases

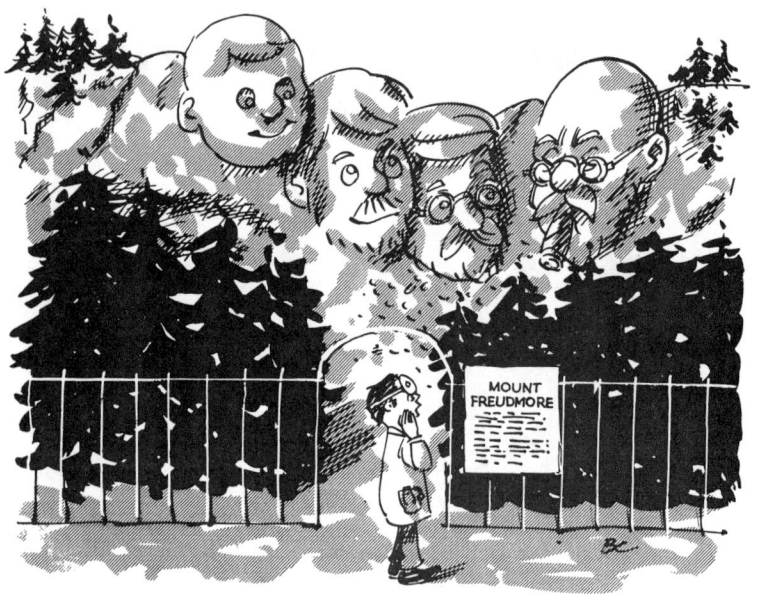

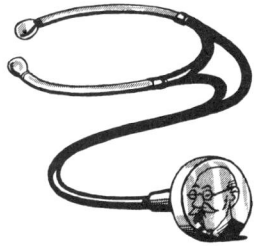

1/ History & Organization of C-L Psychiatry

Introduction

Consultation-liaison (**C-L**) refers to the branch or subspecialty of psychiatry that focuses on the interface between psychological (mental) and somatic (medical) illnesses. C-L psychiatry is an integral part of **psychosomatic medicine**, which involves:

> • the study of the effects of psychological and social factors on physiological functions in the development, course and outcome of illness
> • using a **biopsychosocial** approach in understanding and treating the predisposing, precipitating, perpetuating and preventative (or protective) aspects of illnesses
> Adapted from Lipowski (1984) & Engel (1977)

The main function of C-L psychiatry is to provide clinical services that link mental health professionals to those in other medical specialties (as illustrated below), on both an inpatient and outpatient basis. As a field of scientific endeavor, C-L psychiatry also has education and research components.

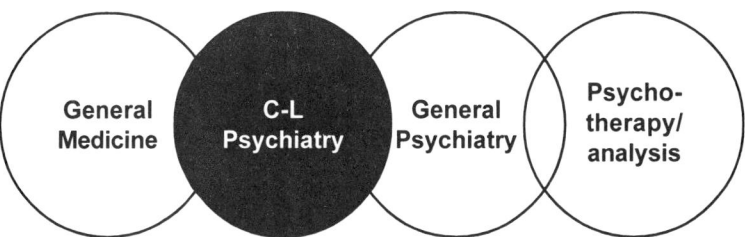

Sigmundoscopy — The Bases

C-L psychiatry can be conceptualized as bridging the gap between illnesses which are entirely physical in nature and those considered to have entirely psychological causes.

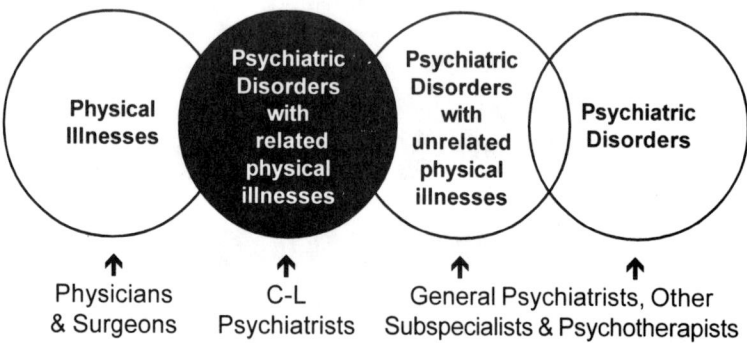

Depending on the availability of clinical resources, some hospitals have psychiatrists who further specialize and offer their services exclusively to areas where the psychosocial aspects of illness are particularly pronounced. The most common services requiring this degree of psychiatric involvement are: Transplantation, Cardiology, Gastroenterology, Oncology and HIV Clinics. The **American Hospital Association (AHA)** estimated in 1984 that almost nine-hundred hospitals offered C-L services.

Noyes (1992) reported on the **Academy of Psychosomatic Medicine (APM)** survey of the 6000 members of the **American Psychiatric Association (APA)** (membership at that time — 36,740) who indicated an interest in C-L psychiatry. It was estimated that about 2,700 psychiatrists (7.5% of the membership) spent at least one-quarter of their time engaged in C-L work, and nearly 1,200 psychiatrists (3.2% of the membership) spent at least half their time involved in C-L activities. The majority of psychiatrists conducted less than one-hundred and fifty inpatient consults per year, though some were referred up to six-hundred per year.

Further, about 3,800 psychiatrists (10.5% of the APA membership) had some affiliation with a C-L service (i.e. involved in conducting consults, educational activities or research).

C-L is the Complete Subspecialty

Psychiatry is a diverse field. Psychiatrists are commonly and unfortunately polarized into being either principally psychopharmacologists (biologically-oriented) or psychotherapists (dynamically-oriented). Both sides have their strengths and weaknesses, proponents and opponents. There are subspecialties within psychiatry (listed later in this chapter) that further narrow the range of patients that some psychiatrists treat.

If there is one quality that does apply to psychiatry as a whole, it is the avoidance of physical examinations and the lack of familiarity with diagnostic tests. Kick (1997), reporting on this observation, states that. . . *as a result, the discipline's claim that it alone is capable of including medical causes of psychiatric syndromes produces a hollow tone to non-psychiatric physicians who observe their practice.*

All psychiatrists have completed medical school, yet the knowledge so acquired tends to play a minimal role in their day-to-day practices. C-L is the subspecialty that ties together all the "factions" of psychiatry as well as keeping its practitioners in touch with medical and surgical practices. C-L psychiatrists require at least a working knowledge of the following areas:

- Psychotherapy
- Forensics
- Addictions
- Neuropsychiatry
- Psychopharmacology
- Geriatric & Adolescent Psychiatry
- Emergency Psychiatry
- Crisis Intervention

In this way, C-L psychiatry is the complete subspecialty. The diagnostic diversity is at least as varied as that encountered on general psychiatry units, with additional skills being required to adapt management plans to patients' physical illnesses. Since the majority of psychiatrists engaged in C-L work do not make this their only avenue of practice, they have the opportunity to enhance their skills in other areas. It is not unusual to have researchers, psychoanalysts or even administrative psychiatrists involved in C-L activities for a portion of their practice.

Sigmundoscopy — The Bases

Langlsey (1988) conducted a survey among psychiatric practitioners and educators regarding their opinions on what skills and knowledge define a specialist in psychiatry. Forty-eight items regarding skills and fifty-one items regarding knowledge were ranked. Those particularly relevant to C-L psychiatry with an agreement of at least 90% are listed below with their rank:

Rank	Skill
1	• conduct a comprehensive diagnostic interview
10	• maintain records including history, mental status exam, physical examination, diagnostic tests and progress notes
11	• conduct crisis intervention
12	• use appropriate laboratory tests, psychological testing and other diagnostic procedures
14	• conduct a comprehensive assessment and develop a management plan for physically or psychosomatically ill patients
15	• conduct brief psychotherapy
16	• develop liaison relationships with other professionals

Rank	Knowledge
2	• differentiate between physical and psychiatric disorders
5	• evaluation and management of psychiatric emergencies
11	• psychiatrically relevant aspects of neurology
12	• psychological aspects of stress, coping, loss, bereavement, etc.
13	• syndromes of importance in C-L psychiatry
14	• indications/contraindications for various forms of psychotherapy
15	• indications/limitations of psychological testing

C-L work requires the greatest breadth of skills and knowledge of all the areas in psychiatry. As an example, consider the range of abilities required to manage the following case:

A sixty-seven year old male with a history of bipolar mood disorder is admitted after a lithium overdose. Because of his high serum lithium level, he is too obtunded to consent to dialysis, which is deemed necessary by the medical consultant. Substitute consent is obtained for this procedure. After recovering from the overdose, he goes into alcohol withdrawal delirium two days later and attempts to leave hospital. After crisis intervention takes place to prevent him from leaving, his status is changed to that of an involuntary patient (due to safety concerns and so he can receive further treatment). He receives medication to treat his withdrawal. Once he recovers from the withdrawal delirium, he requests psychotherapy to help him deal with his "anniversary reaction" to his wife's death.

A Rose By Any Other Name...

Schwab is credited with first using the term "consultation-liaison" in the late 1960's (Mendel & Solomon, 1968). Since this introduction, use of the term has been met with considerable controversy, aptly summed up by Bronheim, quoted in Thompson (1993):

All physicians reserve for themselves the right, honor, and privilege to consult with patients for colleagues. Using the word consultation in our title, irrespective of what specialized knowledge we may have about a particular patient population, even one that no other psychiatrist would want to treat, is exclusionary and fundamentally an insult to our psychiatric colleagues. (p. 259)

Thompson (1993) contacted two-hundred and ten psychiatrists, selected by him, half of whom were prominent educators and/or clinicians who did not primarily practice C-L psychiatry, with the other half from the APM. Recipients were asked to define the role, patient population and expertise possessed by C-L psychiatrists. Their consensus was as follows:

C-L psychiatrists evaluate and treat inpatients and outpatients with significant medical and surgical illness who are also experiencing significant psychiatric symptoms. These patients' symptoms may be due to their medical-surgical conditions, medical-surgical medications, and other treatments (and may be worsened by these factors), and their psychiatric symptoms may be interfering with optimal medical management. (p. 260)

Alternative names for the subspecialty were also solicited. The most common suggestions were:

- Psychosomatic Psychiatry
- Psychiatric Medicine
- Medical Psychiatry
- Medical-Psychiatric Practice
- General Hospital Psychiatry
- Medical-Surgical Psychiatry
- Psychiatry of the Medically-Surgically Ill

The clear favorite was **Medical-Surgical Psychiatry**. This term was considered to be both concise and reflective of the patient population treated, though it was criticized for leaving out other specialties (e.g. Obstetrics-Gynecology (Ob-Gyn)).

Consultation Psychiatry

Although the term **C-L** is usually globally applied to the activities described above, **consultation** and **liaison** in practice encompass separate functions.

Consultation refers to the provision of clinical services for a patient at the request of the primary (non-psychiatric) physician. The consultation involves an interview, followed by the development and implementation of a treatment plan. The aim of the consultation is to answer the clinical question(s) posed by the referring physician, and to assist in the management of this central problem and related issues.

Lipowski (1986, 1996) proposed the following models of consultation, which were established during what he terms the **conceptual development phase** of C-L psychiatry from 1960 — 1975:

> • **Patient-Oriented Consultation** — in which the patient is the main focus of the consultant's inquiry; this type of consultation involves a diagnostic interview, personality assessment, psychosocial data, understanding the meaning of the illness to the patient and determining reactions to past stressors

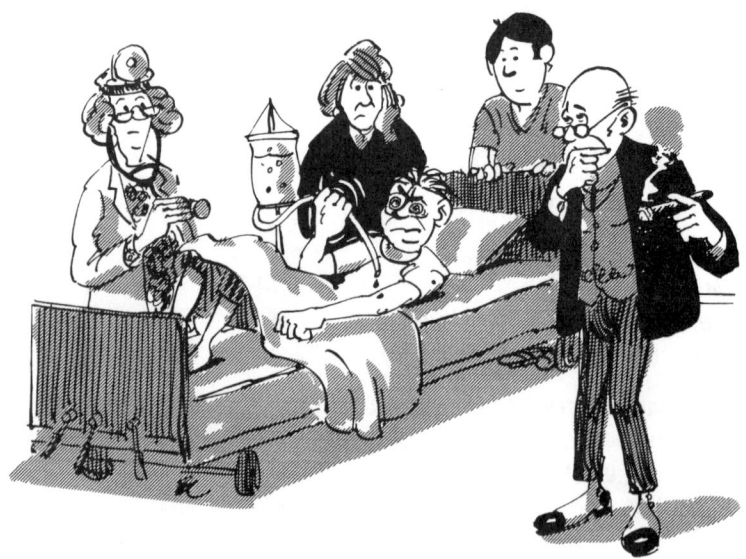

History & Organization of C-L Psychiatry

- **Crisis-Oriented Consultation** — this involves a rapid assessment of the patient's problem(s) and active intervention on the part of the consultant

- **Consultee-Oriented Consultation** — focuses on the needs of the referring source, such as countertransference difficulties, splitting of the staff, disagreement on management, etc.

- **Situation-Oriented Consultation** — one concerned with the interaction between the patient and the clinical team; **Expanded Psychiatric Consultations** involve the patient, friends, family, the clinical team, other consultants, clergy, etc.

The consultation model of service delivery is based on the case method in which the consultee initiates the process. Requests are made once problems have developed and been recognized. In this way, the consultations focus on **secondary prevention** (limiting the development of symptoms after they have developed) and **tertiary prevention** (rehabilitating patients to prevent the recurrence of symptoms). There is no formal, structured teaching of psychiatric principles, though practical, clinical points germane to the particular case may be emphasized.

Consultation services meet the basic or essential clinical needs of referring sources. Many psychiatrists call themselves only "consultation psychiatrists" if they do not provide liaison services.

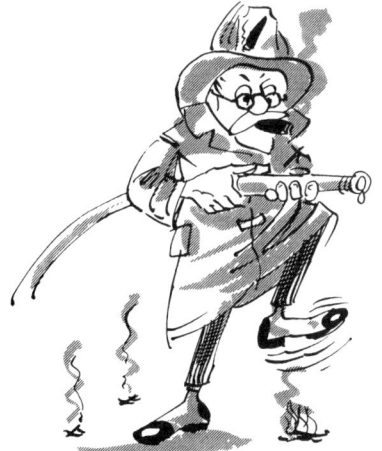
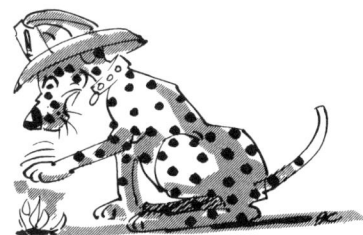

A frequent comparison of the consultation model is that of "putting out fires."

Liaison Psychiatry

Liaison (a French term meaning "to bind") was first used by Billings (1939), and refers to activities that promote an awareness of psychiatric and psychosocial issues in patients' care. These educational contacts can be either formal (e.g. structured teaching rounds) or informal (e.g. a brief review of ego defense mechanisms). Other definitions of liaison are *a linking up or connecting of two or more separate entities, especially military units, so they can work together effectively*, and *an illicit love affair*. Clearly, not all of these aspects fall within the mandate of liaison psychiatry. In general, liaison activities are carried out to:

- increase the attention paid to the psychosocial aspects of a patient's care and to practice **primary prevention** strategies (preventing the development of psychological symptoms)
- educate medical/surgical colleagues about the psychological effects of being ill, and how this affects the speed and extent of a patient's recovery
- help break down the barriers between psychiatry and other specialties by maintaining a presence on their units, being readily accessible to assist, and having expertise helpful both to patients and medical/surgical staff members
- impart basic psychosocial knowledge and to help foster the ability of other physicians in detection and triage techniques
- provide continuing education for non-psychiatrists, and to promote structural changes in medical/surgical settings

The traditional medical model involves the consultation approach, in which an assessment and management plan are provided at the request of the consultee. This is largely a reactive measure. The liaison approach is more proactive, and may involve psychiatrists becoming integrated members of medical or surgical teams. Attendance at rounds and clinics provides regular contact with medical or surgical colleagues. Liaison psychiatrists do not wait for formal consults to be requested — they involve themselves in the care of all patients on a particular service where significant psychiatric issues are identified. Formal teaching is provided in areas relevant to current patients' needs. Liaison activities can also consist of a series of seminars, the topics of which are geared to

History & Organization of C-L Psychiatry

attaining educational goals independent of the ward milieu. Liaison psychiatrists also involve themselves in assisting medical and surgical staff with their reactions to the patients, and to each other (with respect to their clinical work). Education of patients and families regarding psychosocial issues is another commonly requested liaison activity.

Liaison programs often require alternate forms of funding because a significant amount of psychiatrists' time is spent in dealing with the staff instead of patients, a role not typically remunerated by managed care organizations. Due to the time investment in providing liaison services, a single psychiatrist can only offer his or her expertise to a limited number of areas in the hospital. For these reasons, the liaison model is not without its detractors. In addition to the concerns about the time investment and financial support, liaison psychiatrists have been described as being "intrusive" or even "nuisances" on medical/surgical units. For this reason, liaison services are considerably scarcer than consultation services.

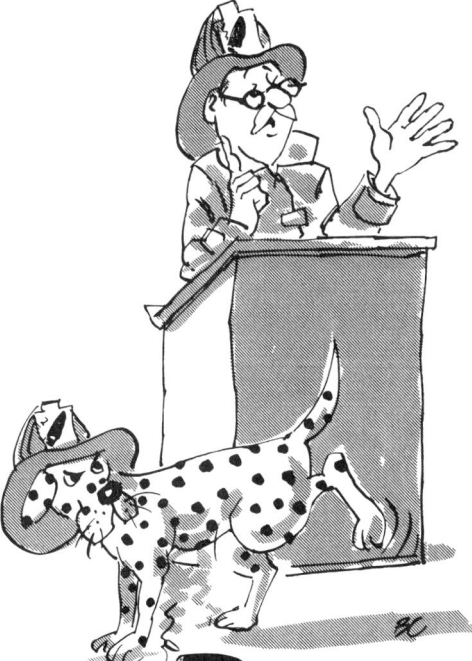

Hospitals that have liaison programs gear them towards units where there is a high likelihood that patients will develop psychiatric disorders (e.g. transplant programs), and often employ mental health professionals other than psychiatrists.

> A frequent comparison of the liaison model is that of lecturing on fire safety.

Despite the gains that can be made in both patient care and educating physicians, liaison activities have generally been declining since the 1980's, mainly due to funding difficulties.

Hackett (1978) expressed pessimism in the overall effectiveness of liaison efforts on medical and surgical wards. In a 1982 lecture to the APM, he said "*It is time for liaison psychiatrists to realize that their goal of converting other physicians to view disease as having a psychosocial as well as a somatic component cannot be accomplished.*"

Rosenbaum & McCarty (1994) observed that the first chapter in the *Handbook of General Hospital Psychiatry* underwent significant changes from the first to the third edition (now fourth edition): the number of pages was halved from fourteen to seven, and the name was changed from "*Beginnings: Liaison Psychiatry in the General Hospital*" to "*Beginnings: Consultation Psychiatry in the General Hospital.*"

Rosenbaum & McCarty (1994) explain the fate of liaison psychiatry in terms of the milieu on medical/surgical wards. In these areas, physicians are faced with the following challenges:

- acquiring and mastering the skills in their own disciplines
- looking after seriously ill patients
- providing care primarily to reduce symptoms
- facilitating discharge from the hospital in a timely manner

They make the cogent point that medical and surgical residents are just as humane and broadminded as psychiatric residents, however given the highly demanding circumstances under which they train, it may be adaptive for them to suppress their humanistic interests (at particular times).

Most hospital psychiatry departments are not able to offer liaison services. However, consultation activities can be quite comprehensive and involve: following patients during their entire stay; family interviews; contacting collateral sources of information (e.g. family doctors, pharmacies); thorough chart reviews, etc.

Psychosomatic Medicine and C-L Psychiatry

The forerunner of American psychosomatic medicine is widely considered to be Benjamin Rush, who said in one of his lectures, *"Man is said to be a compound of soul and body. However proper this language may be in religion, it is not so in medicine. He is, in the eye of the physician, a single and indivisible being, for so intimately united are his soul and body, that one cannot be moved without the other."* (Rush, 1811)

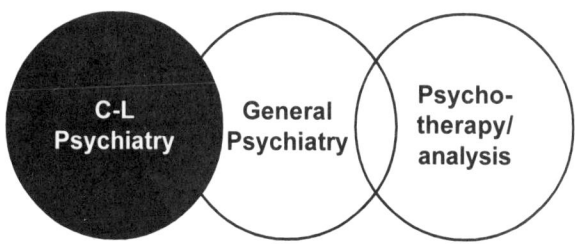

Despite the polarity suggested by the above diagram, the pioneers of C-L psychiatry were psychiatrists who with psychoanalytic training and interests. Though Rush emphasized a holistic view of illness, psychosomatic medicine did not develop in the United States until the 1930's. Most of the presidents of the **American Psychosomatic Society (APS)** between 1942 — 1958 were psychoanalysts (Rosenbaum & McCarty, 1994). The most visible early goal of psychosomatic medicine was to attribute the pathogenesis of specific physical illnesses to unconscious conflicts.

Both psychosomatic medicine and the emergence of general hospital psychiatric units led to the development of C-L psychiatry, which Lipowski (1996) delineated into three main phases:

- **Organizational Phase** (1935 — 1960): formation of discrete C-L services and an evaluation of the usefulness of these activities; expansion of teaching roles
- **Conceptual Phase** (1960 — 1975): focus on the process and conduct of consultations (various models were proposed)
- **Rapid Growth Phase** (1975 — 1980's): NIMH supported the development and expansion of C-L services; major goals were educating primary care physicians and expanding research

A Brief History of Psychosomatic Medicine

Despite the relatively recent use of the term "psychosomatic" and its delineation as a branch of medicine, the concept of unity and a reciprocal relationship between the health of the mind and the health of the body has existed since antiquity.

Ancient societies appreciated that there was a cause-and-effect connection between mind and body. Indeed, illnesses were deemed to be caused by social and emotional factors, and often thought to have magical or religious origins. Accordingly, efforts to treat disease were largely based on such beliefs, and succeeded because of the faith that the afflicted person had in spiritual healers. The power invested by society in such shamans, as well as their interpersonal qualities, were the curative factors in these early "doctor-patient" relationships. Early misconceptions about the human body held that the heart was the center of intellectual ability and that the function of brain was to cool the heart. These views are still popular among some cardiologists.

One of the many lasting contributions from the late Greek/Roman era was the awareness that illness stems from disturbances arising from within the body. Hippocrates, Plato and Aristotle, among many others, recorded observations linking reciprocal effects that the mind and body had on each other. Socrates stated that "*As it is not proper to cure the eyes without the head, nor the head without the body, so neither is it proper to cure the body without the soul.*" While Galen correctly determined that the brain was the center of intellectual and emotional activity, soma and psyche were considered as one during this formative period in medicine.

With the disintegration of ancient Greek and Roman civilizations, the concept of illness reverted back to attributing causation to personal, societal or spiritual causes. Religious factors in particular were considered dominant forces in the etiology of illness (i.e. sinning). Until the Renaissance, religious figures were the ones principally involved in treating sickness.

History & Organization of C-L Psychiatry

Scientific advances led to the discovery that certain illnesses had demonstrable organic findings. Autopsies revealed that organ and tissue changes, rather than those in the spiritual realm, caused or were associated with diseases. The use of the microscope enabled disturbances to be detected on a cellular level. Thus began an era where the cause of illness could be elucidated, pathological findings correlated and remedies sought — which shifted medicine's focus from treating the patient to treating the illness.

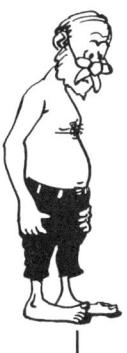

Psychosomatic medicine is concerned "holistically" with the whole patient — the effects of the mind on the body and vice versa.

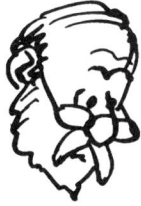

PSYCHE

The study of the psyche became divided — the "mind" by philosophers and the "soul" by theologians. The emotional aspects of illness (both causing and being the result of physical illnesses) are difficult to substantiate objectively because of the high degree of variability from person to person

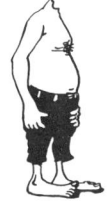

SOMA

Virchow, the founder of modern pathology, stated that "*disease has its origin in disease of the cell*" in that:
• subcellular components are affected by disease, eventually altering cellular structure and function
• tissue and organ changes are observable on micro- and macroscopic levels

Sigmundoscopy — The Bases

In the early 1900's Freud re-established the link between psyche and soma. Josef Breuer, Freud's friend and colleague, described his treatment of a twenty-one-year-old woman (called **Anna O** when the case was published). Her symptoms developed as she nursed her dying father. She suffered from a nervous cough, visual disturbances, paralysis of the right arm, hydrophobia, and experienced visual hallucinations. She also alternated between two levels of consciousness: normality, and another where she regressed to a child-like state, which she called her "naughty states." Breuer noted that when she was in this regressed state, he could at times get her to describe the emotional circumstances surrounding the onset of a symptom, which would later lead to its disappearance. Anna O called this "chimney sweeping" or the talking cure. Breuer called it his cathartic method. For example, her visual difficulties began when she had to squint to hold back her tears when looking at her watch to tell her father the time. Her paralyzed arm stemmed from a daydream in which she visualized a snake about to bite her father, but her arm had gone to sleep because it was resting over the back of the chair and she was unable to reach out and help.

As the patient (her real name was Bertha Pappenheim) improved, it became obvious that she had developed an affection for Breuer (by many accounts it was mutual). Only hours after he had terminated the relationship, he was called back to her bedside to find her in the midst of pseudocyesis (hysterical childbirth). The episode so upset Breuer that he left for a second honeymoon shortly after this event. After much persuading from Freud, he recalled these events after about thirteen years, and the two collaborated on the book, *Studies on Hysteria* (1893 — 1895).

Through the cases of Anna O, **Dora** and others, Freud became interested in the "talking cure" as a treatment. He renewed interest in the doctor-patient relationship as a therapeutic modality. He used the term **transference** (the patient's inappropriate and anachronistic experiencing of the therapist as a significant figure from his or her past) and **countertransference** (the therapist's conscious, emotional reaction to the patient).

History & Organization of C-L Psychiatry

Freud, a neurologist by training, had worked with Charcot in Paris. This had given him first-hand experience with **hysteria**, a condition in which Charcot took a special interest. Freud observed that hypnotic suggestion could cause hysterical (physical) manifestations, which started him thinking about hysteria having a psychological origin. He had developed a special interest in linking hypnosis and neurology, and ultimately psychology to neurophysiology, and called it **Project for a Scientific Psychology**.

Freud was also influenced by Helmholtz, the German physiologist and physicist. Freud's theories have a mechanistic quality to them which borrow from the physical sciences. Initiated through his collaboration with Breuer, Freud developed a theoretical framework for the pathogenesis of hysterical symptoms, based on the idea that such patients suffer from *reminiscences*.

> The patient experienced a past (usually childhood) trauma which was unpleasant and painful.

> The event overwhelmed the patient's ability to deal with it, and is **repressed** into the unconscious; the emotional energy (**affect**) associated with the trauma was strangulated (not expressed).

> The strangulated affect caused nervous excitation, which is converted via unconscious mechanisms into somatic channels (the voluntary nervous system) and expressed in hysterical symptoms.

> Because of the number of psychological events between the original trauma and the hysterical symptom(s), the patient was conscious of only a disguised connection to the event; the hysterical symptom remains symbolically linked to the event/conflict.

> If therapy can bring the event back into consciousness, along with the strangulated affect, the symptoms caused by the unconscious will disappear as the affect is discharged (called **abreaction**).

Freud had now developed a revolutionary concept whereby a purely mental event/agent directly affected physical functions in the body. This theory held considerable appeal because it seemingly described the interrelationship between psyche and soma, and that a form of treatment was efficacious in hysterical conditions. Others sought to expand on this concept and give psychophysiologic explanations for a range of somatic disorders.

In the 1930's, Franz Alexander posited that psychosomatic symptoms developed in organs innervated by the **autonomic nervous system**. Using the **fight-flight** concept developed by Cannon (1915), Alexander reasoned that symptoms could be caused by hyperarousal after exposure to a stressful situation. He did not feel the resulting psychosomatic symptoms had specific psychological meanings, rather they were the result of prolonged tension.

Alexander considered **conversion reactions** to be mediated by the voluntary nervous system. In keeping with Freud's psychodynamic ideas, Alexander also concluded that a conversion (hysterical) symptom was a symbolic representation of the conflict or repressed emotion.

Early workers developed two schools of thought regarding psychosomatic medicine. One group held that specific emotions or personality styles caused particular somatic changes which in turn led to particular diseases. The ensuing school of thought became referred to as the **specificity theories**.

The other main avenue of pursuit, referred to as the **nonspecific theories**, held that generalized stress, tension or anxiety could, over time, initiate the pathogenesis of any of a number of illnesses. Constitutional predisposing factors (e.g. genetic loading, concurrent illness, etc.) in combination with the prolonged stress would determine which condition(s) resulted. The role of certain personality types or emotional stimuli were not considered.

More recent theories are termed **multifactorial** or **multidisciplinary**, which emphasize a more balanced approach.

♦ Specificity Theories

Although these theories have been all but disproven and are often criticized, they were initially met with a good deal of enthusiasm because it was hoped psychiatry could share a predictable and verifiable basis for illnesses with the other fields in medicine. Two key figures involved in specificity theories were Franz Alexander and Helen Flanders Dunbar.

Alexander (1950, 1968) postulated that the use of **ego defenses**, which are unconscious mechanisms that diminish the anxiety accompanying conflict, are linked with the **autonomic nervous system (sympathetic** and **parasympathetic)** and ultimately affect the internal organs (called **organ neurosis**). Alexander proposed specific theories for seven illnesses: essential hypertension, rheumatoid arthritis, thyrotoxicosis, peptic ulcer, ulcerative colitis, bronchial asthma and neurodermatitis. As an example, patients with peptic ulcers were thought to have oral-dependency longings that were frustrated, leading to an impotent rage and the unconscious coexistence of hunger and anger. This conflict became physiologically activated in increased gastric secretions (hydrochloric acid, pepsin, etc.). Experimentally, stressors have been found to increase acid secretion and motility while decreasing bicarbonate secretion. Despite numerous case reports, controlled studies have failed to consistently show that peptic ulcer disease follows stressful life events.

Dunbar (1934, 1936) published her observations on the role of personality factors in some seven-hundred patients with diverse medical problems. In particular, she reported on the way personality influenced the etiology, severity and response to treatment, as well as how it was affected by the illness. For example, she found that patients with hypertension were often psychologically "on guard" and that diabetic patients often had "passive personality traits." Dunbar, having established the APS, has been recognized as the founder of modern psychosomatic medicine. While much of her work was not substantiated over time, she provided an early description of the **Type A Personality** later published by Friedman & Rosenman (1959, 1970).

◆ Nonspecific Theories

The nonspecific aspects of these theories are twofold in that neither individual traits nor particular illnesses are part of these formulations. Additionally, these theories are based more on experimental observation than on psychoanalytic theory.

When an organism is subjected to a stressor, the **autonomic nervous system** becomes activated. This can be manifested in both the **sympathetic branch** (e.g. **flight or fight**) or the **parasympathetic branch**, leading to increased vegetative activity. Kaplan (1980) proposed that there are four reactions to stress:

- normal — awareness is followed by a defensive action
- neurotic — the level of anxiety is so great that the defense becomes ineffective
- psychotic — the "alert signal" is misperceived or ignored
- psychosomatic — the psychic defense fails, so the "alert" is transferred to the somatic systems

The nonspecific theories focus on the effects of chronic stress and how this is translated into somatic dysfunction. In general, organ systems will hyper- or hypofunction in terms of vascularity, motility, secretions, etc. when a person is subjected to stress.

Wolf & Wolff (1943, 1950) observed altered function in gastric and respiratory function. Intuitively, hostility would seem to cause a hyperfunctioning, while fear and sadness would reduce functioning. They concluded that psychosomatic diseases result from attempts to deal with chronically stressful situations. The alterations in physiologic functioning mentioned above are presumed to lead to permanent changes in organ structure and function.

Some theorists incorporated the tenets of **learning theory** in that the protective mechanisms, while initially **unconditioned reactions** to physical stimuli, become conditioned responses to psychological stimuli. This might allow for **symbolization** to occur, in that the physiologic reaction is linked to a psychological stressor (e.g. gastrointestinal disorders developing in obsessive-compulsive personalities).

◆ Multidisciplinary Theories

In order to furnish explanations for the diverse manifestations of psychosomatic illness, current theories take into account a person's constitutional and social factors. The constellation of possible outcomes is determined by the person's genotype. Inherited tendencies may cause a particular organ to become vulnerable, such as a sensitivity to **parasympathetic stimulation** leading to motility disturbances in Irritable Bowel Syndrome. Social factors are also of primary importance in determining the time of onset and severity of many illnesses. Holmes & Rahe (1967) developed a weighted scale of stressors and proposed that a certain level of stress (adding the numbers assigned to individual events) heightened the likelihood of impending illness.

Current research efforts are investigating the modulation of the **immune system** by the central nervous system and the field of **psychoneuroendocrinology** in an effort to delineate mechanisms for psychosomatic responses.

◆ Psychosomatic Points ⊙

- Heinroth, in 1818, was the first to use the term **psychosomatic**, and did so describing the origin of insomnia
- the American Psychiatric Association, in the DSM-I (1952), called these disorders, "psychophysiologic autonomic and visceral disorders;" this was changed to "psychophysiologic disorders" in the DSM-II (1968) and to "psychological factors affecting physical conditions" in the DSM-III (1980)
- some of the specific conflicts considered operative in Alexander's seven psychosomatic conditions were:

• peptic ulcer	dependence vs. independence
• intestinal disorders	riddance vs. retention
• hypertension	suppression of rage and anger
• asthma	an unconscious wish for protection
• thyrotoxicosis	exaggerated fear of death or injury
• rheumatoid arthritis	feelings of inadequacy
• neurodermatitis	craving for physical closeness

Current Psychosomatic Concepts

The terms **psychosomatic** and **psychosomatic medicine** still carry considerable ambiguity. Lipowski (1984) traced the historical references and uses of the these terms, and offers the following definitions:

> • **psychosomatic** — refers to the inseparability and interdependence of psychosocial and biologic (physiologic, somatic) aspects of humankind
>
> • **psychosomatic medicine** — refers to the discipline concerned with **a)** the study of the correlation of psychologic functions, normal or pathologic, and of the interplay of biologic and psychosocial factors in the development, course, and outcome of diseases; and **b)** advocacy of a holistic (or biopsychosocial) approach to patient care and application of methods derived from behavioral sciences to the prevention and treatment of human morbidity.

Lipowski stresses that there have been two enduring aspects of psychosomatic medicine:

> • **the holistic conception** — which refers to the treatment of the whole patient in focusing on emotional/psychologic factors in addition to the somatic/physiologic; this is accounted for in the definition of psychosomatic
>
> • **the psychogenic conception** — which refers to the mental or psychological etiology of an illness

The **psychogenic conception** has caused considerable debate among many workers in the psychosomatic field. Emotions are currently viewed not as solely etiologic agents, but as intermediaries bridging external events and somatic responses. Particularly eschewed is equating the terms *psychogenic* and *psychosomatic*. The above definition of psychosomatic emphasizes the multifactorial understanding of illnesses taking into account biological factors (involving both genetics and current state of health), social circumstances and unique psychological meaning of events. Patients' emotional health has a clear effect on both their somatic

History & Organization of C-L Psychiatry

and psychiatric illnesses. In a very real sense, every illness can be considered as psychosomatic in origin, yet this is rarely emphasized in other medical specialties. Take for example the situation where a patient with an exacerbation of asthma requires admission and is treated with oxygen, bronchodilators, etc. Under these circumstances, psychological precipitants are seldom elucidated. Further, issues such as compliance with medication or concurrent smoking have a large bearing on the illness, but are often addressed only with a "lecture" from the treating team.

Physical medicine specialties often make a sharp distinction between *biological* and *psychosocial factors*. Despite the relevance of psychosocial factors to all illnesses and the repeated calls for such factors to be emphasized in medical training, they are usually relegated to C-L teams to sort out (when these factors are recognized). The most common "psychosomatic" psychiatric conditions for which consults are requested are the following:

Somatoform Disorders

Somatization Disorder	Conversion Disorder	Hypochondriasis
characterized by symptoms which are not due to a recognized medical condition or the effects of a substance, and involve: • pain • gastrointestinal symptoms • sexual symptoms • pseudoneurologial symptoms	characterized by: • deficits in the motor or sensory function • the inability to account for the findings on the basis of a known illness or effects of a substance • adverse psychosocial factors are deemed to be involved in the onset of the illness	characterized by: • an excessive and unreasonable concern with having a serious medical illness despite adequate investigations and reassurance • mininum 6 month duration • the ideas are not of the same intensity as a delusional belief

Consults are frequently requested for two other conditions:
• **Malingering** — the conscious production of symptoms for an obvious gain (called **secondary gain**)
• **Factitious Disorder** — the conscious, volitional production of physical or psychological symptoms in order to assume "the sick role" (secondary gain not obvious)

Psychological Factors Affecting Medical Conditions

Psychological Factors Affecting Medical Conditions (**PFAMC**) is the term used in the DSM-IV (APA, 1994) so that relevant factors are included in the diagnostic nomenclature, coded as follows:

[*Specified Psychological Factor*] Affecting... [*Indicate the General Medical Condition*]

A. A general medical condition (coded on Axis III) is present.
B. Psychological factors adversely affect the general medical condition in one of the following ways:
    (1) the factors have influenced the course of the general medical condition as shown by a close temporal association between the psychological factors and the development or exacerbation of, or delayed recovery from, the general medical condition
    (2) the factors interfere with the treatment of the general medical condition
    (3) the factors constitute additional health risks for the individual
    (4) stress-related physiological responses precipitate or exacerbate symptoms of the general medical condition

The DSM-IV goes on to further specify the major parameters that are subsumed under the term "psychological factors."

Choose name based on the nature of the psychological factors (if more than one factor is present, indicate the most prominent):

• Mental Disorder Affecting... [*Indicate the General Medical Condition*] (e.g., an Axis I disorder such as Major Depressive Disorder delaying recovery from a myocardial infarction)

• Psychological Symptoms Affecting... [*Indicate the General Medical Condition*] (e.g., depressive symptoms delaying recovery from surgery in a patient with cancer; anxiety exacerbating asthma)

• Personality Traits or Coping Style Affecting... [*Indicate the General Medical Condition*] (e.g., pathological denial of the need for surgery in a patient with cancer; hostile, pressured behavior contributing to cardiovascular disease)

• Maladaptive Health Behaviors Affecting... [*Indicate the General Medical Condition*] (e.g., overeating; lack of exercise; unsafe sex)

History & Organization of C-L Psychiatry

• Stress-Related Physiological Response Affecting. . . [*Indicate the General Medical Condition*] (e.g., stress-related exacerbation of ulcer, hypertension, arrhythmia, or tension headache)

• Other or Unspecified Psychological Factors Affecting. . .[*Indicate the General Medical Condition*] (e.g., interpersonal or cultural factors)

Reprinted from the DSM-IV.
© American Psychiatric Association, Washington, DC, 1994
Used with permission.

Both psychosocial and behavioral factors are considered important in every illness. PFAMC is used in cases where the psychological factor(s) is(are) deemed to have a clinically significant effect on the development, course or recovery from a medical condition. Inherent in the use of PFAMC is the temporal association of relevant psychosocial factors. These influences remain speculative and await further clear-cut evidence.

PFAMC is found in the *Other Conditions That May Be a Focus of Clinical Attention* chapter in the DSM-IV. It is coded on Axis I with the accompanying medical condition on Axis III. If present, personality disorders, traits and prominent ego defense mechanisms and mental retardation are coded on Axis II.

Before diagnosing PFAMC, the following conditions must be excluded:

- Substance Abuse, Dependence or Withdrawal States — these entities can be indistinguishable from primary psychiatric disorders
- Adjustment Disorders — are due to an identifiable stressor and can have somatic manifestations (e.g. vegetative symptoms of depression)
- Somatoform Disorders — involve the presence of physical symptoms with no clear organic cause

A detailed presentation of PFAMC can be found in:
   A. Stoudemire, Editor
   Psychological Factors Affecting Medical Conditions
   American Psychiatric Press, Inc., Washington DC, 1995

A Brief History of C-L Psychiatry

There is likely to be little opposition to the statement that psychiatry is the most ostracized of the medical specialties. C-L psychiatrists are often regarded as the "black sheep" of the various subspecialties within psychiatry. Being at the beck and call of other doctors, making recommendations that require approval before implementation, assessing and treating patients on medical-surgical wards and having to constantly deal with variably informed or interested consultees combine to make C-L work a "challenge" that most are happy to forgo. Even within the subspecialty, there are rifts between those who primarily do the "lowly" consults and those involved in the more elegant task of liaison psychiatry (referred to in Murray (1989) as a group of "busy-bodies").

Psychiatry, despite being the earliest distinct specialty,* has been both ideologically and geographically isolated from the rest of medicine. In an address to the American Medico-Psychological Association, Mitchell (1894) accused psychiatrists of being cut off from the mainstream of American medicine by sequestering themselves in "monasteries of the mad."

Separate wards for psychiatric patients date as far back as the 8th century in Muslim history. Asylums were created in Europe somewhere around the 13th century. Such institutions were frequently the sites of torture and other inhumane acts perpetrated in the name of "treatment." With the evolution of medical thought, and the discovery of the nervous system (partly elucidated via autopsies conducted by Morgagni), other theories arose that helped diminish the association of "madness" with evil or sin. Psychological and environmental causes for mental illness were considered in the late 1700's. Pinel, Chiarugi, Tuke and Langermann worked to bring about reforms in asylums in separate countries. Pinel is particularly known for his initiative regarding the moral treatment of the insane.

* **The American Journal of Psychiatry** is the oldest, continuously published medical specialty journal in the United States.

History & Organization of C-L Psychiatry

Originally, in some U.S. hospitals, psychiatric patients were kept on the same units as medical patients. For reasons such as sporadic violence, unpredictability or behavioral disturbances, asylums were created to house the "insane." These institutions, separate from other medical facilities, were usually in rural locations, acerbically described by Shem (1997) as "out of mind, out of sight." Asylums generally functioned under the direction of a superintendent. In 1844, the **Association of Medical Superintendents of American Institutions for the Insane (AMSAII)** was formed. The membership of this organization declined to join the **American Medical Association (AMA)** in 1857. The name was eventually changed to the **American Medico-Psychological Association** in 1892, and finally to the APA.

Initially, neurologists were the specialists called upon to consult on the psychiatric patients who were outside of the asylums. Hysteria, neurasthenia, psychasthenia and psychoneurosis were common ailments for which a neurological opinion was sought. The interplay of various factors shaped the direction of psychiatry. The AMA, in 1870, made psychiatric education a requirement in medical schools. The advent of the hospital being a site of teaching and research in addition to clinical work drew psychiatrists out of the asylums.

It is widely held that the first "consultation" psychiatrist was in fact the eminent neurologist, and co-founder of the **American Neurologic Association (ANA)**, James Putnam. His approach to both treating and understanding illness was influenced by William James, one of the founders of experimental psychology. Another physician trained in neurology, Adolf Meyer, developed a theory of **psychobiology**, which refocused attention on the individual instead of the disease. In particular Meyer advocated an approach based on "total personality reactions" which took into account hereditary, environmental, social and cultural factors.

Though a comprehensive presentation on the history of C-L psychiatry is beyond the scope of this book, an outline of some of the important individuals and events is given in the next section.

Sigmundoscopy — The Bases

◆ Benjamin Rush (died 1813)
Sixteen Introductory Lectures
Bradford & Innskeep, Philadelphia, 1811
Rush held the view that mental and physical illnesses were interrelated in that adverse psychological reactions could be the cause of many diseases; he advocated for the integration of this understanding in medical education. For his early, compassionate and prophetic views, Rush is considered the founder of American psychiatry, and his visage graces the seal of the American Psychiatric Association.

◆ In 1867, the first American medical education course in psychiatric illness was given (Ebaugh, 1944).

◆ John P. Gray
Insanity and Its Relations to Medicine
American Journal of Insanity 25: p. 145 — 172, 1868
In this article, Gray encouraged the inclusion of psychological disorders in the curriculum of medical schools.

◆ J. Montgomery Mosher
A Consideration of the Need of Better Provision for the Treatment of Mental Disease in its Early Stage
American Journal of Insanity 65: p. 499 — 508, 1909
The author was the one who, in 1902, started the first sustained general hospital psychiatry unit in Albany, N.Y. Only a few equivalent units opened around the country in the next two decades.

◆ Adolph Meyer
Psychobiology: A Science of Man
Charles Thomas Publishers, Springfield, IL, 1957
Meyer first used the term **psychobiology** in 1915 to describe the development of an individual in light of his or her environment. This concept centers on "the mind in action" in balancing conscious drives and adaptation to the surroundings. Meyer considered mental functions as part of the whole person, not a separate aspect. He defined mental health as freedom from conflict or friction.

History & Organization of C-L Psychiatry

◆ George W. Henry
Some Modern Aspects of Psychiatry in General Hospital Practice
American Journal of Psychiatry 86: p. 481 — 499, 1929
This landmark paper is widely considered the first description of C-L practice (it must be — it contains no references!), and helped it grow in stature as an important area of psychiatry. Many of Henry's observations are still relevant today:

> • consultees often overlook psychiatric issues and make referrals only after no physical explanation for an illness can be found
> • psychiatrists obfuscate their findings with jargon and instead need to state their formulations in plain language
> • an in-depth interview of the patient is required, as well as the use of all available sources of information
> • treatment needs to be individually formulated
> • observations instead of theories should be the guiding principle in conducting consults

◆ Starting in 1931, Alan Gregg directed over 11 million dollars in grants from the Rockefeller Foundation for the development of psychiatry and its related fields in cities around the country.

◆ Helen Flanders Dunbar et al
Psychiatric Aspects of Medical Problems
American Journal of Psychiatry 93: p. 649 — 679, 1936
Reported on the influence psychological factors had on a wide number of medical conditions, both in terms of etiology and course of the illness.

◆ Edward Billings
Value of Psychiatry to the General Hospital
Hospitals 15: p. 30 — 34, 1941
Billings, considered a pioneer of psychosomatic medicine, established a liaison department at the University of Colorado. He developed a structured three-month rotation for psychiatric residents and a one-month rotation for medical interns. He was one of the first to document the cost savings from liaison activities.

Sigmundoscopy — The Bases

◆ M.R. Kaufman & S.G. Margolin
Theory and Practice of Psychosomatic Medicine in a General Hospital
Medical Clinics of North America 32: p. 611 — 616, 1948
Kaufman developed the model for hospital-based psychiatric services, in particular liaison activities on medical-surgical wards. He was a strong proponent of early indoctrination to psychosomatic concepts for students, residents and other staff members.

◆ Grete L. Bibring
Psychiatry and Medical Practice in a General Hospital
New England Journal of Medicine 254: p. 366 — 372, 1956
She delineated three key areas of clinical activity for C-L psychiatry: differentiating between organic and psychogenic conditions; the use of "psychotherapeutic" medicine using differential approaches to patients; and physician self-awareness

◆ Eugene Meyer et al
Psychiatric Consultations With Patients on Medical and Surgical Wards: Patterns and Processes
Psychiatry 24: p. 197 — 220, 1961
This paper substantially expanded the conceptual basis for C-L and analyzed the interactions in the consultation process.

◆ Z.J. Lipowski, 1967 — 68
Review of Consultation Psychiatry and Psychosomatic Medicine (see references)
This series contains articles detailing the general principles, clinical aspects and theoretical issues in the above areas. Additionally, Lipowski described the organization, scope and function of a C-L service.

◆ 1970's: The NIMH Psychiatry Education Branch supported the development of C-L services nationwide, linked recognition of the importance of psychosocial issues to primary care, and the expertise of C-L psychiatrists in providing education.

◆ 1980's: C-L programs were significantly affected by cutbacks; as of 1985 NIMH training grants were discontinued.

History & Organization of C-L Psychiatry

Abilities of a C-L Psychiatrist

• an expert knowledge of psychiatric disorders, a working knowledge of medical (physical) disorders, and the ability to understand the relationship between the two (**biopsychosocial** orientation)

• able to use varied treatment modalities for medically ill patients (especially in psychopharmacology); provision of short-term psychotherapy is an important aspect of care that was not initially emphasized in early concepts of C-L service

• capable of working in a non-psychiatric setting; able to communicate with physicians, housestaff, nurses, families and patients

• able to discern and accommodate the idiosyncrasies of consultees and specialized units; observant of both the needs of the consultee and the patient; able to respond to all parties in a beneficial manner

• able to gather clinical data from several sources into a coherent summary (formulation) using a biopsychosocial approach to develop and implement a management plan

• able to rapidly obtain and assimilate information, form hypotheses, and make effective interventions; these skills may differ significantly from those required in other areas of psychiatry

• able to elicit pathological findings/diagnostic criteria in interviews and mental status examinations (MSE)

• cognizant of the legal and ethical principles involved in patients' medical care (e.g. competence to consent to treatment, confidentiality, sharing of records, etc.)

• able to interpret basic hematologic, biochemical and neuroimaging results and be knowledgeable in directing further testing (for both medical and psychological aspects)

• being an interested teacher who is capable of passing along useful information to referring sources, as well as teaching nurses, students, psychologists, social workers, etc.

• able to supervise and work with a multidisciplinary team

Qualities of a C-L Psychiatrist

• must wait for others to recognize problems that were potentially obvious at an earlier point (and then await the consult request)

• able to tolerate abuse and rejection from patients who are not cooperative or haven't been informed of consults

• able to admit he or she doesn't know what is wrong and/or has little (or nothing) to offer

• able to tolerate not getting paid for some clinical work

• avoid pretending to be able to magically treat the patient

• constantly monitoring management steps and changing approaches quickly when they are not successful

• able to tolerate criticisms of the specialty (valid and otherwise) from patients and staff alike

• able to tolerate disruptions and to keep a flexible schedule

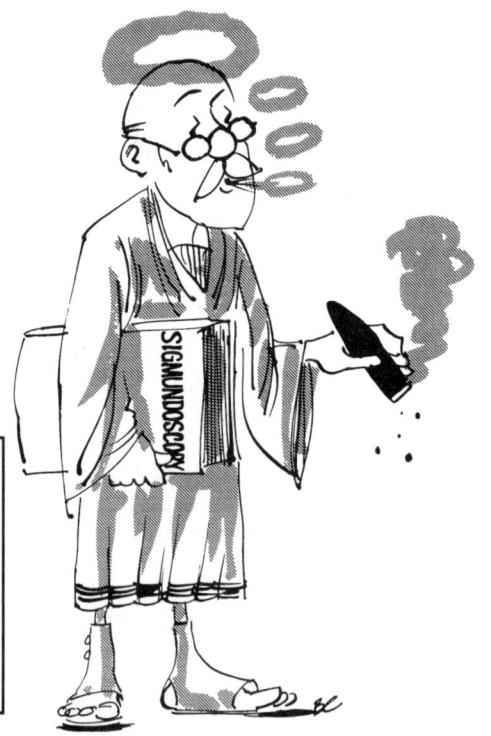

> "The liaison psychiatrist is some form of 20th century masochist, half-deluded and saintly at the same time"
>
> M.H. Greenhill

C-L Education

Education in C-L psychiatry takes place mainly on a postgraduate level. Lectures to undergraduate students are given in some medical schools, and a growing number of introductory textbooks include chapters on C-L psychiatry. It is difficult enough for medical students to master their basic clinical skills, let alone grasp the complex interactions occurring in C-L processes.

In the United States, the **Accreditation Council for Graduate Medical Education (ACGME)** requires psychiatry residents to complete a C-L rotation of at least two months duration. On a practical level, this usually translates into at least a three-month rotation. A C-L exposure is not required of residents by the **Royal College of Physicians and Surgeons of Canada (RCPSC)**, though it is a common practice to split a six-month rotation between Geriatric Psychiatry and a C-L service.

C-L rotations provide valuable experiences for residents. In addition to staying current with medical and surgical treatments, C-L exposures hone residents' skills as psychiatrists. Hayes (1996) notes that consultation exposure provides the opportunity to *". . . do rapid and accurate diagnostic evaluations, understand the implications of other illnesses, treatments, and relationships, advise a primary physician about how to manage the problem, and be available for consultation when things don't go well."*

The development of such skills benefits residents in all aspects of their education and the care they provide. Gains in the following areas are particularly significant:

- emergency room interviews
- oral examinations (e.g. departmental exams, board exams)
- communicating with non-psychiatric physicians (especially the patient's family doctor)
- keeping in mind the need to investigate possible organic causes for psychiatric conditions
- seeing a relatively large number of patients with diverse illnesses within a short period of time

Sigmundoscopy — The Bases

In 1996, Gitlin et al published an article in **Psychosomatics** entitled *Recommended Guidelines for Consultation-Liaison Psychiatric Training in Psychiatry Residency Programs*. These guidelines were the result of a collaborative effort involving all 196 U.S. accredited psychiatry programs over a four-year span, as well as the expertise of members of the APM, **Association for Academic Psychiatry (AAP), American Association of Directors of Psychiatric Residency Training (AADPRT)** and the APA. Up until this publication, only broad objectives for rotations had been discussed. Standards for C-L training programs were presented in Cohen-Cole (1981).

Most programs employ idiosyncratic approaches to C-L training that are primarily influenced by local factors (e.g. the protocols developed by the current education director). Over the time span that C-L has been developing as a subspecialty, there have been no widely accepted standards adopted by general psychiatry residency programs. A summary of the guidelines from Gitlin (1996) is as follows:

A/ Goals of C-L Training
- exposure to a wide variety of patients
- concise interviewing and rapid diagnostic assessments
- determine the impact of illness on psychological functioning
- consider biopsychosocial factors in the etiology of illness
- increasing residents' fund of knowledge
- encourage consultees to consider psychosocial factors
- develop facility with a wide range of interventions

B/ Objectives for Psychiatry Residents in C-L Psychiatry
- *C-L Process* (learning how to interact with consultees; gathering data; writing consultation notes; monitoring progress)
- *Examination Skills* (interviewing medically ill patients; evaluating psychiatric signs and symptoms in physically ill patients; assessing cognitive abilities)
- *Therapeutic Interventions* (determining the effect of the illness and treatment on psychological functioning; use of psychotropic medications in medically ill patients; use of psychotherapies in medically ill patients; functioning as part of a multidisciplinary team)

History & Organization of C-L Psychiatry

C/ Recommended Curriculum Content for C-L Psychiatry Rotations
- Category 1: Essentials for general psychiatrists
- Category 2: Core Knowledge for C-L psychiatrists
- Category 3: Advanced Level Topics

D/ Structure & Integration
- Ideal Rotation (full time block of four to six months duration with participation in one-hundred consultations)
- When to do a C-L Rotation (third or fourth year is optimal)
- Setting for C-L Experiences (general medical hospital)

E/ Faculty Staffing
- Qualified supervisor (board certified, specific expertise)
- Full-time appointment of supervisor to C-L service
- One supervisor for maximum two residents

F/ Teaching and Supervision
- resident able to watch a complete consultation
- resident supervision for at least one complete consultation and in all related aspects of the consultation process
- daily contact with the supervisor
- primary site of supervision is on the medical wards
- supervisor monitoring of resident teaching activities
- residents' notes read and co-signed
- comprehensive and structured didactic teaching
- resident taught how to access medical literature

C-L Bibliographies

M.C. Cremens, L.V. Calabrese, J.L. Shuster & T.A. Stern
The Massachusetts General Hospital Annotated Bibliography For Residents in Training in Consultation-Liaison Psychiatry
Psychosomatics 36(3): p. 217 — 235, 1995

C.F. McCartney, D.L. Evans & W. Richardson
Library Collection of Psychosocial Publications in C-L Psychiatry
General Hospital Psychiatry 7: p. 73 — 82, 1985

J.J. Strain, J.S. Hammer, C. Lewin et al
The Continuing Evolution and Update of a Literature Search Schema for Consultation-Liaison Psychiatry: 1991
General Hospital Psychiatry 13: p. 1 — 62, 1991

C-L Research

Research in C-L psychiatry is a diverse and growing aspect of the field. Some of the major areas of investigation are:

• What percentage of patients with psychiatric difficulties or psychosocial factors affecting their medical illnesses are referred to psychiatrists? Why is this? What factors influence referral rates?

• How common are psychiatric illnesses in medically ill patients?

• What are the common or expectable psychological reactions to physical illness and injury? What are the common or expectable physical complications of psychiatric illnesses and medications?

• What constitutes a normal reaction to an illness? At what point is this process considered pathological?

• In what ways do psychological factors affect physical illnesses? How thorough does the treatment of these factors have to be to optimally benefit patients' recovery?

• How effective are psychiatric consultations in detecting and treating mental illnesses? How can this be increased/optimized? What impact does a consultation have on quality of life, morbidity of physical illnesses, length of stay and overall cost of hospitalization?

• To what extent do consultees follow management recommendations? What can be done to maximize this? Why would they not follow psychiatrists' suggestions?

• Is psychiatry different than other fields in the number of consults requested, or the response to those consults?

• Which treatments are most effective? How can new methods be developed, or current modalities be modified, to improve our usefulness to patients and consultees?

- Demographics of patients referred; most common diagnoses among those referred

- Which services consistently refer patients? Why is this?

- What happens to patients who are identified as requiring psychiatric consultations but are not referred?

- Do C-L services change attitudes towards psychiatry?

- What impact do C-L services make on referral rates?

- How do patients view psychiatric consults?

- Research into psychiatric conditions that commonly present with physical symptoms (i.e. Somatoform, Conversion and Factitious Disorders)

Cohen-Cole (1986) mentions seven key C-L research topics: diagnosis, disease mechanisms, biologic treatments, health services research, psychosocial treatments for medical disorders, epidemiologic issues and education research. He notes that C-L research focuses on clinically significant psychiatric and psychosocial problems in medical/surgical patients. This differs from research in behavioral medicine, which typically looks at life-style or risk factor contributions to medical illnesses.

Weisman (1993) with insights developed from his distinguished career, presents an engaging review of medical research, his varied interests, and his strong desire to see progress in C-L psychiatry. He lists common reasons for avoiding research, and notes that "*C-L psychiatry did not start out nor establish itself as a conduit for research. . . it did not advance as it has because of research in the field. There has been precious small amount of that. It has grown because of its contributions to intelligent patient care.*"

Weisman further states "*Some investigators need microscopes; others telescopes; still others, questionnaires. I think C-L research will progress more rapidly as other methods of investigation develop. . . collaboration with non-psychiatric colleagues is a good way to examine answers that someone else has asked.*"

Funding and Composition of C-L Teams

In the current era of managed care, cost containment, etc., it should come as little surprise that C-L services have also been affected by cutbacks. As described previously, the Rockefeller Foundation financially supported the development of inpatient psychiatric units in general hospitals. Later, the NIMH Psychiatric Education Branch began funding C-L training grants (including fellowships) from the early 1970's to the early 1980's. Since that time, funding for C-L activities has been declining (Koran, 1992).

Cavanaugh (1995) reported the results of a survey of 76 C-L programs across the U.S.:

- 32% of programs experienced a decrease in funding
- 54% reported no changes/stable funding arrangements
- 14% had an increase in funding

Despite these results, in 57% of programs funding was considered to be a major problem, resulting in the reduction or discontinuation of liaison activities in about two-thirds of respondents. Just over half of the programs reported that they were understaffed.

Funding from alternate sources is crucial to the maintenance of an effective C-L service. A good deal of time is spent in activities that do not involve face-to-face contact with patients, which is the major stipulation for reimbursement for clinical services. As will be outlined in later chapters, consultation activities require frequent contact with consultees, housestaff, family doctors, pharmacies, patients' families, etc. Liaison activities involve even less patient contact and are highly dependent on alternate sources of funding. Currently, forty-five programs in the U.S. offer C-L fellowships (they are listed with the APM Guide to Fellowships). All of the institutions offering fellowships were contacted by Strain (1995) and asked about their current funding and level of staffing. The results of this survey are as follows:

- Psychiatry Dept. — 42%
- Hospital — 29%
- Patient Fees — 13%
- Other Dept. — 6%
- Grants — 5%
- Medical School 3%

History & Organization of C-L Psychiatry

The structure and role of a full C-L team is as follows:

C-L Psychiatrists
- supervise the team; in programs with more than one psychiatrist, each one may develop particular interests and divide consults accordingly, or simply alternate seeing new patients

C-L Fellows
- these are physicians who have completed psychiatry residency programs and are seeking additional training to further refine, enhance and expand their skills
- often fellowships involve the opportunity to specialize in particular aspects of C-L work (e.g. HIV or Oncology) and to begin or continue research; also have teaching responsibilities

C-L Residents
- these are physicians who have completed medical school and are taking additional training in psychiatry; a two-month C-L rotation is required in the U.S.
- residents usually perform the majority of the consultation work

Medical Students
- students may have the opportunity to work on C-L teams as part of their clinical clerkship or on elective rotations
- they are generally supervised when with patients and in some cases may only be allowed to observe

Psychologists
- hold an MA or PhD; role in C-L team varies; often involved in psychometric testing, research and liaison activities

Nurses/Nurse Clinicians
- variety of qualifications from RN to PhD; role in C-L team varies; often involved in liaison activities, obtaining collateral information, patient teaching, family meetings

Secretaries on C-L teams play a critical role as they must triage referrals and know the schedules/availability of all the other members. None of the programs reported in Strain (1995) had social workers, but again, he contacted only those with fellowship programs. Social workers play a valuable role on C-L teams, often fulfilling the tasks described for psychologists and nurses.

Outpatient C-L Psychiatry

Outpatient C-L psychiatry has been defined as being an endeavor linking physical care with mental health care (Dolinar, 1993). Pincus (1987) conceptualized five models by which service can be provided between **mental health providers (MHP)** and **primary care providers (PCP)**:

> • **Joint Care Model** — the MHP and PCP work very closely and are in constant communication with each other; an example of this would be a psychiatrist working in a family practice clinic where patients can see both providers in one visit
> • **Consultative Care Model** — the PCP remains the principal provider of care but obtains consultative assistance from the MHP with some form of ongoing communication; an example of this model would be a family doctor who conducts ongoing therapy with a patient while asking a psychiatrist for regular advice on management
> • **Referral Care Model** — here, the MHP is the principal care provider and conducts treatment in relative autonomy; this is the most common model, where patients receive physical care from a physician and a form of therapy from a psychiatrist
> • **Independent Model** and **Autonomous Model** are also described

Dolinar (1993) grouped reports from the outpatient C-L literature and delineated the following categories of clinics providing psychiatric care:

> • **Comprehensive Medicine Clinics** — psychiatric care is provided as part of comprehensive medical care in a medical-type setting
> • **Consultative Clinics** — this is the most common arrangement in which a service is developed primarily to offer consultations to other services, but joint care is rarely given
> • **Psychiatry Clinics** — involve a psychiatric instead of a medical setting, and are primarily geared towards offering treatment instead of consultations

Dolinar (1993) lists twenty-six articles describing the composition and role of clinics providing outpatient services. He notes that studies on outcome and cost effectiveness are lacking.

History & Organization of C-L Psychiatry

Some of the practical advantages and disadvantages in conducting an outpatient C-L service are as follows:

Advantages
- offers consultation to a whole new population of patients
- increases exposure to a wider range of clinical problems
- if working in a multidisciplinary clinic, reduces the stigma of a psychiatric referral; assists with continuity of care
- physical setting is more conducive to interviews (less noise, fewer interruptions, enhanced confidentiality, etc.)
- able to access/arrange for multidisciplinary assessments
- easier to arrange continuing care

Disadvantages
- dependent on referring sources for income; time set aside for consultations (increased availability) can be less remunerative
- "no show" patients can be devastating to a practice because a discrete block of time is scheduled for them, and there is usually no way to recover the time by seeing other patients (which is possible in inpatient settings)
- lack of ward milieu where consultees have easier access to psychiatrists (out of sight — out of mind); do not have the chance to hear about patients who would benefit from consultation
- documentation accompanying outpatients is likely to be less complete than a hospital chart
- being "too available" can decrease the stature of psychiatrists in comparison to other specialties

Further educational advantages for residents and fellows are outlined in Epstein (1993).

Sullivan (1993) points out that outpatient C-L initiatives often face the added difficulty of struggling for both funding and acceptance from patients. He suggests that a multidisciplinary clinic is the ideal venue for outpatient C-L activities, in particular due to the enhanced collegiality with other specialists and reducing the stigma of psychiatric referrals.

With medical care moving more and more toward shortened lengths of stay and outpatient management, there is likely to be an increased demand for C-L services outside of inpatient units.

C-L Practice Guidelines

Gitlin (1996) stated that "*training standards and procedures are often handed down from one C-L director to the next, or brought in with a new director from his/her previous training setting.*" This also tends to occur with practice standards, as until recently there were no comprehensive guidelines for C-L services. Such guidelines would be helpful because of the complex nature of the patients and problems seen on medical/surgical units:

- there are significant rates of psychiatric problems among patients who are physically ill
- the presence of a psychiatric illness usually negatively affects the response to treatment and prognosis of the physical condition(s)
- comorbid psychiatric and physical conditions increase the costs of treatment (including length of inpatient hospitalization)
- the involvement of C-L psychiatrists has been demonstrated to improve patient outcomes and reduce costs

Bronheim (1998), under the auspices of the APM, outlined comprehensive practice guidelines for C-L services. He states that "*These guidelines are not intended to delineate universal, professionally mandated regulations and actions. Instead they are meant to serve as an outline for training and knowledge that are generally necessary to guide the clinician's approach to the patient.*" The proposals set forth by Bronheim (1998) are meant to complement the **APA Practice Guidelines for Psychiatric Evaluation of Adults** (1995).

The aspects of C-L psychiatry for which Bronheim (1998) details guidelines are as follows:

Qualifications of Consultants
- Training & Skills Assessment (includes a comprehensive list of the abilities and functions necessary to run a C-L service)

The Consultation Process
- Indications for Consultation
- Problems Commonly Leading to Consult Requests (a comprehensive list is provided)

- provision for Emergency Assessments
- Components of the Psychiatric History required in consultations
- information required for the Consultation Note
- Diagnostic Testing and Consultation
- provisions for Follow-up Visits, Outpatient Follow-Up, Referral and Signing Off (terminating treatment of the patient)

Interventions
- Psychotherapy
- Pharmacotherapy and Other Somatic Therapies
- Constant Observation and Restraint

Medico-Legal Aspects
- Competency Evaluations
- Involuntary Psychiatric Commitment
- Transfer to Psychiatry Inpatient Units
- Ethical Considerations

Administrative Issues
- Data Collection and Quality Control

Education
- Supervision of Trainees

Special Situations
- Child & Adolescent Consults

Journals
- a list of key sources of C-L literature is provided

Textbooks
- principal texts in the field are listed

Reference Database
- the reference for a literature database is given

Societies
- the key organizations in C-L psychiatry are the **Academy of Psychosomatic Medicine** and the **American Psychosomatic Society**

C-L as a Subspecialty

C-L has yet to achieve official recognition as a psychiatric subspecialty. Currently, there are four such recognized subspecialties in the U.S.: Child & Adolescent, Geriatric, Addiction and Forensic Psychiatry. The RCPSC makes an added qualification available in Child & Adolescent Psychiatry.

The **American Board of Medical Specialties (ABMS)** is the parent organization of the medical specialty boards including the **American Board of Psychiatry & Neurology (ABPN)** and gives final approval to subspecialty designations. They require that an acceptable subspecialty have:

- a strong scientific knowledge base
- learned societies
- journals dedicated to the field
- training programs
- a positive impact on training programs

A strong case can be made for C-L psychiatry being eligible for subspecialty status:

- one-quarter of practicing psychiatrists have some involvement with a C-L service
- C-L is the major activity for 3% of psychiatrists
- sixteen journals (domestic and international) are geared towards publishing C-L literature
- hundreds of books and thousands of articles have been published, giving a knowledge base at least as extensive as the currently recognized subspecialties
- almost fifty C-L programs offer fellowships in the U.S.
- C-L education and experience is a residency requirement in the U.S.
- the ABPN Part I exam (written) tests basic C-L knowledge
- the types of patients typically seen by C-L psychiatrists are not regularly treated by general psychiatrists or the other subspecialties

The case for subspecialty approval has been endorsed by the APA, which was a request of the ABPN. The APA has affirmed the importance of C-L becoming a recognized subspecialty.

History & Organization of C-L Psychiatry

Furthermore, the three cardinal aspects of C-L psychiatry will all benefit from C-L being an added qualification:

Patient Care
- it has been estimated that up to 50% of patients with physical illnesses develop a psychiatric disorder that interferes with the provision of optimal medical care
- typically about 2% of hospital inpatients receive psychiatric consultations
- psychiatric involvement has been shown to lessen symptom severity and reduce the costs of treatment

Education
- added qualification may lead to the development of more C-L Fellowship positions
- many academic institutions will not fund fellowships unless they lead to certification by a nationally recognized organization
- the establishment of more fellowships will mean more emphasis on C-L in psychiatry residencies and medical schools
- without subspecialty status, there is no accrediting body to establish and maintain teaching standards

Research
- general psychiatrists cannot be expected to stay at the forefront of the clinical work done in C-L
- collaboration with specialists from other fields demands knowledge which is beyond that of a general psychiatrist

McKegney (1991) noted the diverse skills required by C-L psychiatrists, with facility being required in the following areas: geriatric psychiatry, neuropsychiatry, substance abuse, psychopharmacology and medicolegal psychiatry. He proposes that C-L is rather a "supraspecialty" that warrants a *Certificate of Added Qualification*. There is little in the literature to oppose official C-L subspecialty status. Muskin (1988) suggests that (further) fragmentation of the profession may occur with granting subspecialty status. While he argues that there are potent financial and political motives for subspecialization, he does not indicate that C-L fails to meet the core ABMS requirements.

Future of C-L Psychiatry

Emerging from psychobiology, general hospital psychiatry and psychosomatic medicine, C-L psychiatry is now in its seventh decade in the U.S. It provides clinical, research and education activities linking psychiatrists to other medical specialties.

◆ **Clinical Service**
C-L services fill a vital role in patient care in general hospitals and outpatient clinics. Patients who suffer from comorbid psychiatric and physical illnesses generally have a lowered response to treatment, a poorer prognosis, and incur greater health care costs. Involving the services of a C-L team is the principal way in which interventions are made to reverse these outcomes. C-L services provide a major, and in some cases, the only link to other specialties within hospitals. This affiliation can be very helpful politically, and gives C-L an optimistic long-term outlook. Having C-L designated as an official subspecialty of psychiatry will help ensure its long-term viability.

◆ **Education**
Gitlin (1996) recommends an increase in the duration of C-L rotations to three months in recognition of the critical role this experience plays in any branch of psychiatry. Given that the detection of medical illness as a causative factor in mental illness is a crucial role of the psychiatrist, this increase would be time well spent.

Kick (1997) proposed a curriculum for medical training in psychiatry residencies. He points out that *"though psychiatrists have remained aligned with medicine. . . training programs do not encourage the application of physical assessment as a part of psychiatric practice."*

◆ **Recruitment**
Psychiatry, already one of the least popular career choices for graduating medical students, has been declining even further in enrolment in recent years (Zaimes, 1994). C-L experiences are optimal in demonstrating the need for, and effectiveness of, psychiatrists in the care of patients from all specialties.

History & Organization of C-L Psychiatry

General References

American Psychiatric Association
Diagnostic and Statistical Manual of Mental Disorders, Fourth Edition
American Psychiatric Association, Washington, D.C., 1994

E.G. Billings
Liaison Psychiatry and Intern Instruction
Journal of the Association of American Medical Colleges: 14, p. 375 — 385, 1939

N.H. Cassem, Editor
Handbook of General Hospital Psychiatry, Fourth Edition
Mosby Yearbook, St. Louis, 1997

S.A. Cohen-Cole, H.A. Pincus, A. Stoudemire et al
Recent Research Developments in Consultation-Liaison Psychiatry
General Hospital Psychiatry 8: p. 316 — 329, 1986

G.L. Engel
The Need for a New Medical Model: A Challenge for Biomedicine
Science 196: p. 129 — 136, 1977

M.H. Greenhill
The Development of Liaison Programs, in G. Usdin, Editor
Psychiatric Medicine
Brunner-Mazel, New York, 1977

T.P. Hackett & N.H. Cassem, Editors
Handbook of General Hospital Psychiatry
C.V. Mosby, St. Louis, 1978

T. P. Hackett
Liasion Psychiatry: Fixture or Fantasy (Invited Lecture)
Academy of Psychosomatic Medicine, November, 1982

S.D. Kick, M. Morrison & R.G. Kathol
Medical Training in Psychiatry Residency: A Proposed Curriculum
General Hospital Psychiatry 19: p. 259 — 266, 1997

D.G. Langsley & J. Yager
The Definition of a Psychiatrist: Eight Years Later
American Journal of Psychiatry 145: p. 469 — 475, 1988

Z.J. Lipowski
What Does "Psychosomatic" Really Mean? A Historical and Semantic Inquiry
Psychosomatic Medicine 46(2): p. 153 — 171, 1984

Z.J. Lipowski
Consultation-Liaison Psychiatry: The First Half Century
General Hospital Psychiatry 8: p. 305 — 315, 1986

Z.J. Lipowski
History of Consultation-Liaison Psychiatry, in
Textbook of Consultation Psychiatry
J.R. Rundell & M. G. Wise, Editors
American Psychiatric Press, Inc., Washington D.C., 1996

Sigmundoscopy — The Bases

D.R. Lipsitt
Use and Abuse of Psychiatric Consultants (lecture)
Meeting of General Hospital Psychiatrists, Boston, Oct. 1972

F.P. McKegney & R.M. Beckhart
Evaluative Research in Consultation-Liaison Psychiatry
General Hospital Psychiatry 4: p. 197 — 220, 1982

R. Noyes Jr., T. Wise & J. Hayes
Consultation-Liaison Psychiatrists: How Many Are There and How Are They Funded?
Psychosomatics 33(2): p. 123 — 127, 1992

M. Rosenbaum & T. McCarty
The Relationship of Psychosomatic Medicine to Consultation-Liaison Psychiatry
Psychosomatics 35(6): p. 569 — 573, 1994

B. Rush
Sixteen Introductory Lectures
Bradford & Innskeep, Philadelphia, 1811

J.J. Schwab
Consultation-Liaison Training Program, in W.M. Mendel & P. Solomon, Editors
The Psychiatric Consultation
Grune & Stratton, New York, 1968

J.J. Strain
The Development and Practice of Liaison Psychiatry, in
Consultation-Liaison Psychiatry: Current Trends and New Perspectives
Grune & Stratton, New York, 1983

T.L. Thompson II
Should We Shift the Name for "Consultation-Liaison" to "Medical-Surgical" Psychiatry, "Psychiatry in Medicine and Surgery" or Some Other Term?
Psychosomatics 34(3): p. 259 — 264, 1993

References for Psychosomatic Section

F. Alexander
Psychosomatic Medicine
Norton, New York, 1950

F. Alexander, T.M. French & G.H. Pollock
Psychosomatic Specificity, Volume 1: Experimental Study and Results
University of Chicago Press, Chicago, 1968

J. Breuer & S. Freud (J. Strachey, translator/editor)
Studies on Hysteria, in The Standard Edition of the Complete Works of Sigmund Freud
Volume 2, Hogarth Press, London, England, 1955
Originally published 1893 — 95

W.B. Cannon
Bodily Changes in Pain, Hunger, Fear and Rage
Appleton, New York, 1915

History & Organization of C-L Psychiatry

W.B. Cannon
The Wisdom of the Body
W.W. Norton, New York, 1932

C.L. Coe
Psychosocial Factors and Immunity In Nonhuman Primates: A Review
Psychosomatic Medicine 55: p. 298, 1993

H.F. Dunbar
Physical Mental Relationships in Illness: Trends in Modern Medicine and Research As Related to Psychiatry
American Journal of Psychiatry 91: p. 541 — 562, 1934

H.F. Dunbar, T.P. Wolfe & J. McK. Rioch
Psychiatric Aspects of Medical Problems
American Journal of Psychiatry 93: p. 649 — 679, 1936

M. Friedman & R.H. Rosenman
Association of Specific Overt Behavior Pattern With Blood and Cardiovascular Findings: Blood Cholesterol Level, Blood Clotting Time, Incidence of Arcus Senilis, and Clinical Coronary Artery Disease
JAMA 169: p. 1286, 1959

M. Friedman, S. Byers & R.H. Rosenman
Coronary-Prone Individuals (Type A Behavior Pattern): Some Biochemical Characteristics
JAMA 212: p. 1030, 1970

D.L. Herzig & K.R. Pelletier
**Psychoneuroendocrinology: Toward A Mind-Body Model
A Critical Review: Advances**
J. Inst. Adv. Health 5: p. 27, 1988

T. H. Holmes & R.H. Rahe
The Social Readjustment Rating Scale
Journal of Psychosomatic Research 11: p. 213, 1967

H.I. Kaplan & H.S. Kaplan
A Historic Survey of Psychosomatic Medicine
Journal of Nervous & Mental Disorders 124: p. 546, 1956

H.I. Kaplan, in
Comprehensive Textbook of Psychiatry, Third Edition
William & Wilkins, Baltimore, 1980

Z.J. Lipowski
What Does The Word "Psychosomatic" Really Mean? A Historical and Semantic Inquiry
Psychosomatic Medicine 46(2): p. 153 — 171, 1984

H.E. Sigerist
A History of Medicine, Volume 1
Oxford Press, New York, 1951

Sigmundoscopy — The Bases

S. Wolf & H.G. Wolff
Human Gastric Function
Oxford University Press, New York, 1943

H.G. Wolff
Life Stress and Bodily Disease: A Formulation
Res. Nerv. Ment. Dis. 29: p. 1059, 1950

References for C-L History Section

F.G. Ebaugh
The History of Psychiatric Education in the U.S. from 1844 to 1944
American Journal of Psychiatry 100: p. 151 — 160, 1944

Z.J. Lipowski
**Review of Consultation Psychiatry and Psychosomatic Medicine
I. General Principles**
Psychosomatic Medicine 29: p. 153 — 171, 1967

Z.J. Lipowski
**Review of Consultation Psychiatry and Psychosomatic Medicine
II. Clinical Aspects**
Psychosomatic Medicine 29: p. 201 — 224, 1967

Z.J. Lipowski
**Review of Consultation Psychiatry and Psychosomatic Medicine
III. Theoretical Issues**
Psychosomatic Medicine 30: p. 394 — 422, 1968

S.W. Mitchell
Address Before the 50th Annual Meeting of the American Medico-Psychologic Association
J. Nerv. Mental Dis. 21: p. 413 — 473, 1894

G. Murray
The Liaison Psychiatrist As Busy-Body
Annals of Clinical Psychiatry 1: p. 265 — 268, 1989

J.M. Quen
**Asylum Psychiatry, Neurology, Social Work and Mental Hygiene:
An Exploration in Interprofessional History**
Journal of the History of Behavioral Sciences 13: p. 3 — 11, 1977

J.J. Schwab
Consulation-Liaison Psychiatry: A Historical Overview
Psychosomatics 30(3): p. 245 — 254, 1989

S.Shem
Mount Misery
Fawcett Books, New York, 1997

History & Organization of C-L Psychiatry

References for Education Section
S.A. Cohen-Cole, J. Haggerty & D. Raft
Objectives for Residents in Consultation Psychiatry: Recommendations of a Task Force
Psychosomatics 23: p. 699 — 703, 1981

D.F. Gitlin, B.A. Schindler, T.A. Stern, S.A. Epstein, R.M. Lamdan et al
Recommended Guidelines for Consultation-Liaison Psychiatry Training in Psychiatry Residency Programs: A Report From the Academy of Psychosomatic Medicine Task Force on Psychiatric Resident Training in Consultation-Liaison Psychiatry
Psychosomatics 37(1): p. 3 — 11, 1996

J.R. Hayes
C-L Psychiatry Residency Training Guidelines: Another Milestone
Psychosomatics 37(1): p. 1— 2, 1996

References for Research Section
S.A. Cohen-Cole, H.A. Pincus, A. Stoudemire, S. Fiester et al
Recent Research Developments in Consultation-Liaison Psychiatry
General Hospital Psychiatry 8: p. 316 — 329, 1986

J. Dimsdale
Challenges, Problems, and Opportunities in C-L Research
Psychiatr. Medicine 9: p. 641 — 648, 1991

F.P. McKegney & R.M. Beckhardt
Evaluative Research in C-L Psychiatry: Review of the Literature: 1970 — 1981
General Hospital Psychiatry 4(3): p. 197 — 218, 1982

A.D. Weisman
Avoiding Research in Consultation-Liaison Psychiatry
Psychosomatics 34(6): p. 469 — 477, 1993

References for Funding and Composition Section
S. Cavanaugh & J. Milne
Recent Changes in Consultation-Liaison Psychiatry
Psychosomatics 36(2): p. 95 — 102, 1995

L. Koran
Funding Consultation-Liaison Psychiatry Via Medicare Screening
General Hospital Psychiatry 14: p. 7 — 14, 1992

J.J. Strain, M. Easton & G. Fulop
Composition and Funding: Consultation-Liaison Psychiatry Services
Psychosomatics 36(2): p. 113 — 121, 1995

References for Outpatient Section

L.J. Dolinar
A Historical Review of Outpatient Consultation-Liaison Psychiatry
General Hospital Psychiatry 15: p. 363 — 368, 1993

S.A. Epstein & J.J. Gonzales
Outpatient Consultation-Liaison Psychiatry: A Valuable Addition to the Training of Advanced Psychiatry Residents
General Hospital Psychiatry 15: p. 369 — 374, 1993

J.J. Gonzales
Outpatient Consultation-Liaison Psychiatry: An Unfulfilled Promise?
General Hospital Psychiatry 15: p. 360 — 362, 1993

H.A. Pincus
Patient-Oriented Models for Linking Primary Care and Mental Health Care
General Hospital Psychiatry 9: p. 95 — 101, 1987

M. Sullivan
Psychosomatic Clinic or Pain Clinic: Which Is More Viable?
General Hospital Psychiatry 15: p. 375 — 380, 1993

References for Practice Guideline Section

American Psychiatric Association
Practice Guidelines for Psychiatric Evaluation of Adults
American Journal of Psychiatry 152(suppl.): p. 65 — 80, 1995

H.E. Bronheim, G. Fulop, E.J. Kunkel, P.R. Muskin, B.A.Schindler, W.R. Yates et al
The Academy of Psychosomatic Medicine Practice Guidelines for Psychiatric Consultation in the General Medical Setting
Psychosomatics 39(4/suppl.): p. S8 — S30, 1998

D.F. Gitlin, B.A. Schindler, T.A. Stern, S.A. Epstein, R.M. Lamdan et al
Recommended Guidelines for Consultation-Liaison Psychiatry Training in Psychiatry Residency Programs: A Report From the Academy of Psychosomatic Medicine Task Force on Psychiatric Resident Training in Consultation-Liaison Psychiatry
Psychosomatics 37(1): p. 3 — 11, 1996

J. Gruman & T.N. Wise
Clinical Guidelines: Now or Never
Psychosomatics 36(6): p. 519 — 521, 1995

A. Stoudemire, H. Bronheim & T.N. Wise
Why Guidelines for Consultation-Liaison Psychiatry?
Psychosomatics 39(4/suppl.): p. S3 — S7, 1998

References for Subspecialty Section

M. Blumenfeld
Subspecialization in Psychiatry is Necessary
Psychosomatics 29(2): p. 153 — 154, 1988

F.P. McKegney, M.A. O'Dowd, C.E. Schwartz & R.M. Marks
A Fallacy of Subspecialization in Psychiatry: C-L Is a Supraspecialty
Psychosomatics 32(3): p. 343 — 345, 1991

P.R. Muskin
Subspecialization in Psychiatry May Fragment the Profession
Psychosomatics 29(2): p. 155 — 156, 1988

C.B. Robinowitz & C.C. Nadelson
Consultation Liaision Psychiatry as a Subspecialty
General Hospital Psychiatry 13: p. 1 — 3, 1991

T.L. Thompson II
Some Advantages of Consultation-Liaison (Medical-Surgical) Psychiatry Becoming an Added Qualification Subspecialty
Psychosomatics 34(4): p. 343 — 349, 1993

T.N. Wise & C.V. Ford
Subspecialization at the Crossroads
Psychosomatics 32(2): p. 121 — 123, 1991

References for Future of C-L Section

D.F. Gitlin, B.A. Schindler, T.A. Stern, S.A. Epstein, R.M. Lamdan et al
Recommended Guidelines for C-L Psychiatry Training in Psychiatry Residency Programs: A Report from the Academy of Psychosomatic Medicine Task Force on Psychiatric Resident Training in Consultation-Liaison Psychiatry
Psychosomatics 37(1): p. 3 — 11, 1996

R.J. Goldberg & A. Stoudemire
The Future of Consultation-Liaison Psychiatry and Medical-Psychiatric Units in the Era of Managed Care
General Hospital Psychiatry 17: p. 268 — 277, 1995

S.D. Kick, M. Morrsion & R.G. Kathol
Medical Training in Psychiatry Residency: A Proposed Curriculum
General Hospital Psychiatry 19: p. 259 — 266, 1997

T.N. Wise, C.W. Schmidt Jr., & J.R. Hayes
Reengineering Consultation-Liaison Psychiatry
Psychosomatics 37(2): p. 91— 92, 1996

J.M.S. Zaimes & T.L. Thompson II
Opportunities for Consultation-Liaison (Medical-Surgical) Psychiatrists to Enhance Residency Recruitment
Psychosomatics 35(5): p. 423— 426, 1994

Sigmundoscopy — The Bases

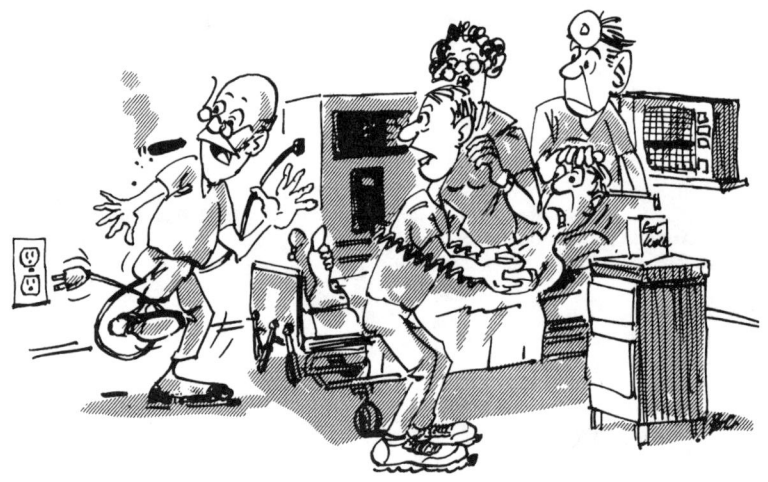

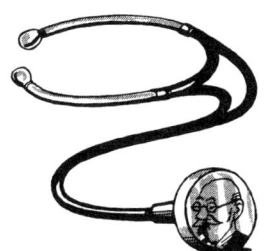

2/ Use & Usefulness of C-L Psychiatry

Psychiatry faces a greater stigma than any other medical specialty. This bias comes from both the public and health care professionals. Steinberg (1994) notes that among physicians, ambivalence towards psychiatry and its practitioners begins in medical school or earlier. He goes on to state that this ambivalence often develops into a bipolar level of expectation regarding psychiatric consultation – either physicians expect too little and don't refer their patients, or expect too much and become disappointed (and as a result stop referring their patients).

The aspects of psychiatry that foster such an ambivalent view are often readily apparent. Many psychiatrists view themselves as having either a "biological" or "psychosocial" orientation, with fervent justification of their practices and the opinion that the "other side" is misguided. In decades past, psychiatrists generated unrealistic expectations about the usefulness of certain treatments (e.g. psychoanalysis), which may well have disappointed referring physicians. It is difficult to gauge the efficacy of psychiatric treatments for a number of reasons:

- improvement happens slowly and may be apparent after only months or years; consultees rarely receive progress updates
- it is difficult to quantify patients' improvement for statistical analyses
- few psychiatric conditions are cured, most are controlled
- many conditions have an episodic course and recur

Sigmundoscopy — The Bases

Because psychotropic medications are generally used to treat target symptoms, a patient's progress can be monitored through a structured set of inquiries (e.g. sleeping patterns, presence of hallucinations). Progress in psychotherapy is more difficult to gauge. Steinberg (1994) addresses this as follows:

At the end of a successful psychotherapy, patients may function better at work, in relationships and in their ability to enjoy recreational pursuits. They may feel better. They may deal with their problems more constructively; this is different from not having problems. None of this implies they will be new people.

C-L and Emergency Psychiatry bring mental health professionals into the greatest degree of contact with medical and surgical colleagues. It is these capacities that practical, effective and timely interventions can be made which make a positive impact on both patient care and our colleagues' impression of psychiatry.

The ultimate utility of psychiatric consults is decided by our customer – the referring physician. Psychiatrists may have a different view than consultees regarding what constitutes a successful consultation outcome:

Medical Consultee ☺	**Psychiatric Consultant** ☹
• patient no longer causing a disturbance on the floor	• alcohol withdrawal delirium under control, but patient refuses Rehab.
• patient transferred to psychiatry inpatient unit, freeing up a bed	• while medically stable, the patient hasn't spoken about the overdose
• patient asked for and received a prescription for antidepressant medication	• tolerability and efficacy of need to be determined; some risk of suicide or induction of a manic episode

In order to run a successful C-L service, psychiatrists must respond to the needs and expectations of their customers, even if this involves addressing the symptoms or surface manifestations of a disorder instead of treating the underlying causes.

Use & Usefulness of C-L Psychiatry

Consultation Requests

Consults are most commonly requested for the following reasons:

◆ **Affect or Mood Changes**
- e.g. depression, anxiety, hostility, irritability, euphoria, etc.

◆ **Behavioral Problems**
- agitation or impulsivity; aggression towards self or others
- demanding to leave the unit; refusing treatment
- crisis intervention (non-violent); chemical or physical restraint

◆ **Capacity Determinations and Forensic Issues**
- capacity consent to treatment (informed consent)
- ability to manage finances or make a Will (testamentary capacity)
- involuntary hospitalization
- ethical issues

◆ **Coping With Medical Illness**
- difficulty accepting diagnosis and/or treatment
- psychological factors affecting medical conditions (PFAMC)
- issues regarding terminal illness (e.g. pain, bereavement, dying)
- maladaptive reaction to illness (e.g. excessive denial, counterphobic attitude, acute stress disorder, posttraumatic stress disorder)
- difficulty interacting with staff members

◆ **Diagnostic Evaluation**
- veracity of complaints (e.g. investigate the possibility of Factitious Disorder, Malingering or a Somatoform Disorder)
- diagnostic evaluation of psychological complaints

◆ **Factors Related to Personal or Psychiatric History**
- sexual abuse; child abuse; elder abuse
- personality disorders
- substance use disorder
- monitoring patients with pre-existing psychiatric disorders even if there are no acute issues (i.e. increasing consultees' comfort level)

◆ **Mental Status Changes**
- e.g. delirium, dementia, psychosis, etc.

◆ **Treatment**
- psychotherapy, pharmacology or other (e.g. ECT)
- transfer of care to an inpatient unit or outpatient program (e.g. resuscitated and detoxified after an overdose)

Sigmundoscopy — The Bases

Depending on the expertise and interests of individual departments, requests from specialized care centers, such as hemodialysis, oncology or prenatal units can be accommodated.

Sections in Chapter One outlined the abilities and qualities characteristic of C-L psychiatrists. While these sections give a general overview, the list on the previous page details the specific problems that consultees will ask to be solved. A number of the capabilities required in these situations are unique to C-L psychiatry, falling beyond the range of expertise found in most general psychiatrists. McKegney (1991) suggests that rather than a "subspecialty" of psychiatry, C-L is a "supraspecialty" due to the breadth of expertise and skills it demands. He goes onto say that:

Clearly, the C-L psychiatrist is the general psychiatrist most experienced in the broad range of problems found in medical settings. If one mental health professional is to be called upon. . . it would seem most efficient to consult a C-L psychiatrist. One call from the consultee to a C-L psychiatrist makes available the broadest range of subspecialty expertise within psychiatry. . . Without the primary care C-L psychiatrist, the consultees would be forced to call upon a wide range of subspecialty psychiatrists, assuming that the consultee internists and surgeons would be able to define the problem clearly enough to identify and call the proper subspecialty consultant.

Consultees deem consultations useful when their expectations are met by the actions of C-L teams. For this reason, it is crucial to obtain clear direction from consultees about their reasons for referring patients, and specifically what type of assistance they seek. In every consultation, there is the opportunity to refine the referring physician's knowledge of how C-L can be helpful to them.

Steinberg (1994), in considering the high rates of divorce, substance abuse and suicide among health care professionals, points out that C-L staff are in a prime position to be of assistance directly to our colleagues. While in many cases this would result in a referral to a therapist who is not acquainted with the individual seeking help, the visibility and reputation of the C-L staff can ease the reluctance colleagues often have in seeking therapy.

Prevalence of Psychiatric Illness

The NIMH completed the **Epidemiologic Catchment Area (ECA)** study in 1980 (Regier, 1988). The results revealed a point prevalence of 15.4% for community residents who met the criteria for one or more DSM-III conditions up to one month prior to the interview. These disorders were distributed as follows:

• Anxiety Disorders	7.3%
• Mood Disorders	5.1%
• Substance Use Disorders	3.8%
• Cognitive Disorders – severe	1.3%
• Schizophrenia	0.6%
• Antisocial Personality Disorder	0.5%
• Somatization Disorder	0.1%

When the five sites involved in the study continued to collect data over the course of one year, it was found that 28.1% of the total population experienced symptoms of sufficient severity to meet DSM-III diagnostic criteria for one or more disorders. Interestingly, only 52% of this population received medical assistance, and of those treated, only 40% received care from a mental health professional (21% of the total population). The figure of 28.1% corresponds to results reported in Goldberg (1980) of a 25% prevalence of psychiatric morbidity in a random community sample.

The percentage of medically ill patients who have comorbid psychiatric illness has been estimated to range from 30 – 65% (Lipowski, 1967; Lipowski, 1975; Moffic, 1975; Goldberg, 1980).

Levenson (1992) screened a group of consecutively admitted medical patients with instruments measuring anxiety, depression, confusion and pain. Of the 1,541 patients included in the study, 741 (48%) had high test scores, which would be a reasonable basis for requesting a psychiatric referral. It is a common experience to see the following features documented on medical charts:

- psychiatric diagnoses recorded in personal histories
- psychiatric medications prescribed
- progress notes indicating ongoing psychosocial difficulties

Sigmundoscopy — The Bases

Despite these indicators that primary physicians have an awareness that psychiatric issues influence patients' care, in most cases consultations are not requested.

The percentage of medical inpatients actually referred for psychiatric consultation ranges from 2 – 12%. Psychiatric departments offering strictly consultation services typically see 1– 3% of medical inpatients, while those offering liaison services can see up to 7 – 10% (Lipowski, 1967; Craig, 1982; Popkin, 1983; Huyse, 1993).

Population	Intervention
Estimated Psychiatric Morbidity in the Community ~25%	Public Education and Screening
↓	
Total Psychiatric Morbidity in General Hospital Inpatients 30 – 65%	Medical Education and Screening
↓	
Total Psychiatric Morbidity in General Hospital Inpatients Recognized by Primary Physicians 10 – 25%	Psychiatric Liaison Activities
↓	
Psychiatric Referral Rate for General Hospital Inpatients 2 – 12%	Psychiatric Consultation

Local and process variables can play dominant roles in determining rates of referral. Local variables are often not easily amenable to change, as they are based on personality factors and/or attitudes towards psychiatry. Process variables are the features of an individual consultation that leave an impression on consultees and affect future referral rates.

Local Variables
• relationships between the psychiatric consultants and referring physicians
• certain specialists and/or specialties place less emphasis on psychosocial factors

Process Variables
• the speed and thoroughness with which consults are carried out
• clear, consistent documentation and communication with the referring source

Characteristics of Patients Referred

The psychiatric diagnoses of patients referred for consultation across three studies were as follows:

Diagnosis	Study 1	Study 2	Study 3
• Adjustment Disorder	25.5%	15%	13%
• Anxiety Disorders	4.5%		2%
• Eating Disorder	1.0%		
• Mood Disorder	22.0%	10%	8%
• Organic Brain Syndrome	20.0%	43%	37%
• Personality Disorder	5.5%		
• Schizophrenia	2.0%		4%
• Somatoform Disorder	4.0%	5%	3%
• Substance Use Disorder	9.5%	8%	11%
• None/Other	3.0%	12%	18%

[1] Wise (1987), [2] Huyse (1993), [3] Huyse (1990)

The four conditions most frequently diagnosed across these studies were: Adjustment Disorders, Mood Disorders, Organic Brain Disorders and Substance Use Disorders. These can be among the most difficult disorders for psychiatrists to treat in consultation situations (e.g. antidepressants usually take from two to six weeks to become effective; delirium is often associated with a poor prognosis; addictive behavior is very difficult to alter).

There may well be a selection bias in that psychiatrists are requested to see patients with disorders that are difficult to treat, especially in the time-limited capacity of a consultation. Referrals may not be requested until complications in patients' medical treatment have developed as a result of their psychiatric problem. There are considerably more patients who could benefit from psychiatric services than are referred. Included in this population are patients with conditions that are potentially easier to treat and would increase the likelihood of demonstrating the usefulness of psychiatric consults. This needs to be kept in mind when reviewing the literature on the cost-effectiveness of C-L activities.

The Effects of Psychiatric Comorbidity

Intuitively, it seems reasonable to assume that patients who suffer from both physical and psychiatric illnesses incur greater health costs and have a less optimistic prognosis for their conditions. An unfortunate relationship between physical and psychiatric conditions can exist in that they perpetuate one another:

Effects of Psychiatric Illness on Physical Illness
- compliance with treatment may be lessened (e.g. patients may have cognitive deficits that prevent a full understanding of the illness, or may have an indifferent attitude towards treatment)
- risk factors such as poor diet, lack of exercise, obesity, smoking, etc. may be more difficult to control

Effects of Physical Illness on Psychiatric Illness
- the stress of somatic illnesses can cause relapses or recurrences of some psychiatric illnesses (e.g. a schizophrenic patient develops a psychotic episode due to an ICU stay)
- treatment of medical conditions can cause some psychiatric illnesses (e.g. steroid-induced psychosis) or worsen pre-existing ones (beta-blockers triggering recurrent depression)

The issue of the effects of psychiatric comorbidity has not received a lot of attention. Sararvay (1994a), in an excellent review of the world literature from 1980 to 1992, found only twenty-six published reports with many having serious methodologic flaws, such as:

- lack of statistical analyses
- no control group
- small sample sizes
- unclear diagnostic criteria
- using the primary physicians' psychiatric diagnoses
- not controlling for the severity of physical or psychiatric illnesses
- study design type (e.g. cross-sectional or retrospective)
- using the presence of a psychiatric consult as the main or sole indicator of psychopathology

Unfortunately, there was considerable variation in the type of comorbid psychiatric illnesses studied. The majority of reports looked only at cognitive dysfunction. Other studies considered mood disorders, substance abuse (alcohol), anxiety disorders and personality features.

In total, twenty of twenty-six articles (~80%) found a statistically significant association between increased **length of stay (LOS)** and psychiatric comorbidity. This finding remains consistent when only the more methodologically sound studies are considered (i.e. prospective studies using control groups and detailed analyses). Of those that did not yield this result, two showed an increase in LOS, but failed to reach statistical significance. Most of the studies not supporting this association had the smallest sample sizes.

The effects of psychiatric comorbidity were found to be an increased LOS and greater use of health care resources after discharge. The strongest association was found for the following illnesses: impaired cognition (delirium and dementia), mood disorders (depression) and personality variables (disorders).

Saravay (1996) conducted a study looking at medical rehospitalization rates over a four-year span in patients with psychiatric comorbidity. He used the **Symptom Checklist 90 (SCL – 90)** as a screening instrument, which measures psychopathology on nine subscales. After controlling for potentially confounding variables, it was found that patients with cognitive impairment, depression and high levels of hostility or interpersonal sensitivity had increased rates of rehospitalization.

Saravay (1994b) makes the apt observation that process research needs to be conducted on how it is that psychiatric disorders actually make an impact on LOS and the cost of medical care (i.e. what is the actual mechanism by which LOS becomes increased).

Outpatient studies have reported that patients with comorbid psychiatric disorders use more health care resources (Katon, 1994), have greater disability (Smith, 1994) and more frequent hospitalizations (Swartz, 1991) compared to those with only physical illnesses. In summarizing these findings, Saravay (1994b) states: *Taken as a whole. . . outpatients and inpatients with psychiatric disorders in the general medical sector use more services, increase the cost of health care, and are more functionally disabled than patients with medical illness only.*

The Effects and Benefits of Psychiatric Interventions

A/ Conceptual Aspects

Billings (1941) reported that C-L services provided for medical inpatients reduced their LOS by almost half, which provided a significant cost reduction considering that the per diem rate for hospitalization was $4. Since then, the economic impact of C-L interventions has been receiving more formalized attention.

C-L is the area of psychiatry most vulnerable to funding cuts, but has the greatest opportunity to provide effective treatments, and to be able to demonstrate this through outcome studies. Saravay (1994b) highlights the paradox that there is growing literature showing:

- psychiatric comorbidity increases health care utilization, and
- C-L activities are effective interventions, both for decreasing patients' symptoms and the costs of treatment

yet points out that these findings have had a limited impact on the financial support for C-L activities. In order to demonstrate the usefulness of C-L psychiatry, the APA established a task force, who in working together with a branch of the NIMH, have undertaken rigorous research studies on cost-effectiveness.

The APM, as the Organization of C-L Psychiatry, seeks not only to facilitate research on outcome studies, but also to secure funding for fellowships and to encourage appropriate reimbursement for clinical activities (i.e. that third-party payors' fee schedules remunerate physicians adequately for these services).

The type and quality of studies being conducted has an impact on the degree to which planners, policy makers, administrators and insurance company executives will be persuaded by the results. Pincus (1984) defines the following types of studies:

Cost-Benefit Analysis (CBA): compares the costs and effects of an intervention using the same measure to gauge the results (usually monetary); studies of this type allow a comparison of dissimilar programs

Cost-Effectiveness Analysis (CEA): compares the costs and effects of an intervention, but the results are measured in different units (for example costs may be measured in time or money while results are expressed in terms of quality of life, reduction of disability or other social judgments); CEA studies are useful in comparing interventions with identical objectives

Cost Efficiency Studies: an analysis of a single program conducted to optimize its interventions

Cost-Offset Study: methodologically weak studies (e.g. anecdotal, retrospective or prospective that don't control for illness severity); these constitute the majority of early reports in which cost reduction was seen as a welcome side effect of the primary intervention of treat mental illness

Further information on study design can be found in Pincus (1984) and Lyons et al (1985).

Lyons et al (1985) indicate that C-L research has two main aims; assessing the efficacy of psychiatric treatments and the cost-effectiveness of these interventions. Accurate measurements of treatment cost and treatment success are crucial to obtain in order to be able to interpret study data. The authors point out that there are costs beyond actual treatment that need to be considered in a CEA, such as loss of productivity and other social factors. In some cases, costs are merely transferred from inpatient to outpatient programs, as in the case of an early or premature discharge. Furthermore, many patients are treated in a variety of settings and costs may be tallied only for one institution.

Treatment effectiveness cannot be gauged only by outcome because level of functioning after an intervention is clearly related to that existing beforehand. Ultimately, a good measure of effectiveness has the following qualities:

- high inter-rater reliability
- sensitive to change
- measures something which is directly related to the effectiveness of an intervention

For example, a study looking at the effectiveness of consultations in terms of which recommendations are followed could meet the first two criteria. However, such a study would not be able to meet the third criterion, because there is no measure of whether the implemented recommendations actually helped patients.

Cohen-Cole (1991) stipulated that three criteria must be met in order to be able to demonstrate the cost-effectiveness of C-L interventions:

- psychiatric disorders must be associated with an increase in medical utilization and cost
- interventions must be able to effectively treat psychiatric conditions (reducing symptom severity)
- medical utilization and its associated costs must be reduced from the baseline concurrent with, or following, the clinical therapeutic changes

The first point was addressed in the previous section by Saravay (1994b) where 89% of studies with a sample size of at least one-hundred-and-ten showed a statistically significant increase in LOS in medical/surgical patients with comorbid psychiatric conditions.

Psychiatrists have been grappling with the second point in order to prove the efficacy of treatment interventions. Issues such as the efficacy of psychotherapy and the necessity of longer-term varieties has been studied extensively in recent years.

The third point presents the greatest challenge for C-L psychiatry in the current climate of cost containment, managed care and health care reform. Guggenheim (1984) stated that:

. . . if a psychiatric intervention not only diminishes the degree of anxiety or anguish but also cuts down the length or cost of a hospital stay, so much the better.

This article, along with Strain (1981), was written as NIMH funding was being withdrawn from C-L programs. These authors were among the first to herald the need to demonstrate that psychiatric interventions were both clinically and economically effective.

B/ Studies from the Literature

◆ *Levitan & Kornfeld, 1981*

This is a frequently cited article involving liaison activities on an orthopedic ward. Patients undergoing surgery (who were not referred for consultation) were divided into an experimental group (who received liaison services) and a control group (who did not). The study found a decrease in LOS of twelve days and that twice as many patients in the experimental group were able to return home instead of requiring placement (e.g. in a nursing home). An almost 20:1 cost saving was projected over the course of one year.

Pincus (1984) lauds the study as meeting strict cost-effectiveness criteria. While many clinical variables were accounted for in the analysis, Pincus points out that the overall availability of nursing home beds and possible changes in health care policies during the study interval were two confounding variables. Strain (1991) enumerates several other factors (e.g. staffing alterations) that could also have affected the results.

◆ *Strain et al, 1991*

This article also reports on a population of patients receiving surgery for hip replacement. The authors point to ten methodological confounds in the Levitan & Kornfeld study and sought to eliminate these from their calculations. This study compared patients on two different wards for two consecutive years. In the first year, patients were referred on a consultation basis, which acted as a baseline or control group. In the second year, a psychiatric liaison service was instituted. This service involved interviewing every consenting patient and offering a treatment plan for psychiatric conditions, weekly "ombudsman" rounds to discuss select cases, and weekly nursing/discharge rounds. At one site, the LOS was decreased by 2.2 days (statistically significant) and at the other it was decreased by 1.7 days (barely missing statistical significance). For the site showing the statistically significant reduction in LOS, the projected savings were almost nine times greater than the cost of the liaison service (which would have been financially self sufficient if the visits were actually billed).

◆ *Strain et al, 1994*
Strain describes a study by Hammer in which patients were screened at the time of admission (the Social-Risk Program) as to whether they were at high risk for requiring psychosocial intervention. This survey found that early identification of high-risk patients shortened the onset C-L activities by 1.2 days (from 4.8 days to 3.6 days) which in turn decreased the average LOS by 6% (a statistically significant finding). The calculated benefit of the Social-Risk Program was $48 saved for each $1 spent.

◆ *Levenson et al, 1992*
This study screened general medical inpatients for the presence of high levels of depression, anxiety, confusion and pain, on the assumption that psychiatric consultation would reduce health care utilization (and cost) both during and after hospitalization. Patients with high screening scores were given a consultation irrespective of whether it was requested by the primary physician. The consultations lasted on average 1.3 hours; only about 10% of these patients received further visits. When the severity of illness was factored into the data analysis, the results showed that patients with high screening scores used more hospital resources, but the psychiatric consultation failed to show any difference in either inpatient costs or post-hospitalization utilization of resources.

Strain (1994) outlines several factors that impede the study of the cost-benefit and cost-effectiveness of C-L activities:

- psychosocial factors are usually identified late in the course of an admission, leaving less time to show the effects of psychiatric interventions
- in many cases, psychiatric recommendations are only partly implemented, which obscures an analysis of effectiveness
- it is extremely difficult, if not impossible, to tell if a psychiatric disorder is caused by a medical illness (physical reaction), a psychological reaction to a medical illness, or occurs independently of medical illness (but has a concurrent presentation)
- there are no suitable instruments to measure the severity of medical illness in patients with comorbid psychiatric conditions
- there are so many confounding variables that it is extremely difficult to conduct random, controlled, double blind studies

The Consequences of Overlooking Psychiatric Problems

In all patients, there are psychosocial variables that affect the course and prognosis of an illness. The statistics quoted earlier in this chapter, along with the tenets of psychosomatic medicine, could justify psychiatric involvement with most, if not all patients. Zimmer (1974) estimated that 12% of patients admitted to medical units were for psychosocial issues. Glass (1978) estimated to figure to be closer to 18%.

When psychiatric referrals are not requested or liaison activities are not conducted, patients either receive treatment from non-psychiatric physicians or receive no treatment at all. Steinberg (1980) found evidence to support a psychiatric consultation in twenty-nine of fifty charts he reviewed, indicating that psychosocial factors were at least recorded by medical/surgical staff. In some cases, psychiatric problems are missed (and hopefully detected by another physician). In other cases, physicians interested in psychiatric issues may wish to treat patients themselves.

Schurman et al (1985) found visits to non-psychiatric physicians for psychiatric reasons to be distributed as follows: Family Physicians 87%; Internists 7.3% and Surgeons 4.2%. Patients were more likely to visit physicians than psychiatrists when they had complaints of sleep disturbances, psychosexual disorders or substance-related problems (including alcohol and tobacco).

Physicians were much more likely than psychiatrists to conduct physical examinations and order diagnostic investigations. Physicians were much less likely to perform an MSE than psychiatrists (6% vs. 30%) or to engage in psychotherapy (25% vs. 96%). Office visits with physicians averaged just under twenty minutes, whereas psychiatrists spent almost forty-five minutes. While physicians were more likely to prescribe psychotropic medications than were psychiatrists (78% vs. 35%, respectively), Wells (1994) stated in treating depression, 40% of patients seen in primary care settings were given subtherapeutic antidepressant doses.

Medical Illness in Psychiatric Patients

One of the many benefits of being involved in C-L activities is the continual reminder of the importance of physical illnesses in psychiatry. Afinson et al (1992), in summarizing other studies, reported that up to 80% of psychiatric inpatients had significant physical illnesses. Koryani (1979) found that in almost half of psychiatric inpatients, their family physicians were unaware of these medical illnesses. In two-thirds of cases, the medical illness was deemed to significantly affect the psychiatric illness, and in one-fifth of cases it was deemed to be the cause. Afinson et al (1992) addresses the issue of laboratory testing to screen for illnesses in psychiatric patients. He reminds us that the history is the most useful means for diagnosing physical conditions, followed by the physical exam and lastly laboratory testing. While there can be a large yield of abnormal results, only about 4% are clinically significant. The following battery can detect over 90% of medical disorders: thorough history, complete physical and neurological examinations; SMA-34 blood chemistry, EKG, urinalysis and sleep-deprived EEG. An algorithm is provided by Sox (1989).

Summary

• the referring source is the ultimate judge of the usefulness of a consultation

• many, if not the majority, of medically ill patients have psychiatric diagnoses or psychosocial issues affecting them, yet the majority of patients suitable for psychiatric consultation are not referred

• often, the most difficult or challenging patients/situations are the ones for which consultations are requested

• liaison activities make a significant difference in the attitude towards psychiatry and the number of referrals made; these activities also change the types of problems for which consults are requested

• educating our colleagues about psychiatric illnesses increases their awareness and sensitivity to patients' psychosocial issues

• patients with comorbid psychiatric and physical disorders are more functionally disabled and have higher treatment costs; the time-limited manner in which patients are seen limits a fuller evaluation of the usefulness and cost-effectiveness of C-L psychiatry

References

T.J. Afinson & R.G. Kathol
Screening Laboratory Evaluation in Psychiatric Patients: A Review
General Hospital Psychiatry 14: p. 248 – 257, 1992

E.G. Billings
The Value of Psychiatry to the General Hospital
Hospitals 15: p. 30 – 34, 1941

S.A. Cohen-Cole, E.F. Howell, J.E. Barnett et al
Consultation-Liaison Research: Four Selected Topics, in F.K. Judd, G.D. Burrows & D.R. Lipsitt, Editors
Handbook of Studies on General Hospital Psychiatry
Elsevier, New York, 1991

T.J. Craig
An Epidemiological Study of a Psychiatric Liaison Service
General Hospital Psychiatry 4: p. 131 – 137, 1982

R. Glass, M. Mulvihill, H. Smith et al
The 4 Score: An Index for Predicting a Patient's Non-Medical Hospital Days
American Journal of Public Health 8: p. 751 – 755, 1978

D.P. Goldberg & P. Huxley
Mental Illness in the Community: The Pathway to Psychiatric Care
Tavistock, London, England, 1980

F.G. Guggenheim
Cost Effectiveness and Consultation Psychiatry: Reflecting On and In Economic Terms
General Hospital Psychiatry 6: p. 171 – 172, 1984

F.J. Huyse, J.J. Strain & J.S. Hammer
Interventions in Consultation-Liaison Psychiatry
Part I: Patterns of Recommendations
General Hospital Psychiatry 12: 213 – 220, 1990

F.J. Huyse, J.S. Lyons & J.J. Strain
The Sequencing of Psychiatric Recommendations: Concordance During the Process of a Psychiatric Consultation
Psychosomatics 34(4): p. 307 – 313, 1993

W. Katon & J. Gonzales
A Review of Randomized Trials of Psychiatric Consultation-Liaison Studies in Primary Care
Psychosomatics 35(3): p. 268 – 278, 1994

E.K. Koryani
Morbidity and Rate of Undiagnosed Physical Illness in a Psychiatric Clinic Population
Archives of General Psychiatry 36: p. 414 – 419, 1979

J.L. Levenson, R.M. Hamer & L.F. Rossiter
A Randomized Control Study of Psychiatric Consultation Guided by Screening in General Medical Inpatients
American Journal of Psychiatry 149(5): p. 631 – 637, 1992

Sigmundoscopy — The Bases

S.J. Levitan & D.S. Kornfeld
Clinical and Cost Benefits of Liaison Psychiatry
American Journal of Psychiatry 138(6): p. 790 – 793, 1981

Z. Lipowski
Review of Consultation Psychiatry and Psychosomatic Medicine II: Clinical Aspects
Comprehensive Psychiatry 16: p. 201 – 224, 1967

Z. Lipowski
Psychiatry of Somatic Diseases: Epidemiology, Pathogenesis, Classification
Comprehensive Psychiatry 16: p. 105 – 124, 1975

J.S. Lyons, J.S. Hammer, T.N. Wise & J.J. Strain
Consultation-Liaison Psychiatry and Cost-Effectiveness
General Hospital Psychiatry 7: p. 302 – 308, 1985

G.P. McGuire, D.L. Julier, K.E. Hawton et al
Psychiatric Morbidity and Referral on Two General Medical Wards
British Medical Journal 1: p. 268 – 270, 1974

F.P. McKegney, M.A. O'Dowd, C.E. Schwartz & R.M. Marks
A Fallacy of Subspecialization in Psychiatry: C-L Is a Supraspecialty
Psychosomatics 32(3): p. 343 — 345, 1991

H. Moffic & E. Paykel
Depression in Medically Ill Patients
British Journal of Psychiatry 126: p. 346 – 353, 1975

H.A. Pincus
Making the Case for Consultation-Liaison Psychiatry: Issues in Cost-Effective Analysis
General Hospital Psychiatry 6: p. 173 – 179, 1984

M.K. Popkin, T.B. Mackenzie & A.L. Callies
Consultation-Liaison Outcome Evaluation System
Archives of General Psychiatry 40: p. 215 – 219, 1983

D.A. Regier, J.H. Boyd, D.S. Rae, J.D. Burke, B.Z. Locke et al
One-Month Prevalence of Mental Disorders in the U.S.; Based On Five Epidemiolgic Catchment Area (ECA) Sites
Archives of General Psychiatry 50: p. 85, 1988

S.M. Saravay & M. Lavin
Psychiatric Comorbidity and Length of Stay in the General Hospital: A Critical Review of Outcome Studies
Psychosomatics 35(3) p. 233 – 252, 1994a

S.M. Saravay & J.J. Strain
APM Taskforce on Funding Implications of Consultation-Liaison Outcome Studies
Psychosomatics 35(3): p. 227 – 232, 1994b

S.M. Saravay, S. Pollack, M.D. Steinberg, B. Weinschel & M. Habert
Four-Year Follow-Up of the Influence of Psychological Comorbidity on Medical Rehospitalization
American Journal of Psychiatry 153(3): p. 397 – 403, 1996

Use & Usefulness of C-L Psychiatry

R.A. Schurman, P.D. Kramer & J.B. Mitchell
The Hidden Mental Health Network
Archives of General Psychiatry 42: p. 89 – 94, 1985

T. Sensky
The General Hospital Psychiatrist: Too Many Tasks and Too Few Roles?
British Journal of Psychiatry 148: p. 151 – 158, 1986

G.R. Smith
The Course of Somatization and Its Effects on Health Care
Psychsomatics 35(3): p. 263 – 267, 1994

H.C. Sox, L.M. Koran & C.H. Sox et al
A Medical Algorithm for Detecting Physical Illness in Psychiatric Patients
Hosp. Comm. Psychiatry 40: p. 1270 – 1276, 1989

H. Steinberg, M. Torem & S.M. Saravary
An Analysis of Physician Resistance to Psychiatric Consultation
Archives of General Psychiatry 37: p. 1007 – 1012, 1980

P.I. Steinberg
What Psychiatry Offers Medicine
Annals of the RCPSC 27(5): p. 283 – 286, 1994

J.J. Strain
Clinical and Cost Benefits of Liaison Psychiatry
American Journal of Psychiatry 138: p. 1630 – 1637, 1981

J.J. Strain, J.S. Lyons, J.S. Hammer, M. Fahs, A. Lebovits, P.L. Paddison et al
Cost Offset Form a Psychiatric Consultation-Liaison Intervention With Elderly Hip Fracture Patients
American Journal of Psychiatry 148(8): p. 1044 – 1048, 1991

J.J. Strain, J.S. Hammer & G. Fulop
APM Taskforce on Psychosocial Interventions in the General Hospital Inpatient Setting
Psychosomatics 35(3): p. 253 – 262, 1994

M. Swartz, R. Landerman, L. George, D. Blazer & J. Escobar
Somatization Disorders, in L.N. Robbins & D. Regier, Editors
Psychiatric Disorders in North America
Free Press, New York, 1991

K.B. Wells
Depression in General Medical Settings: Review of Three Health Care Policies for Consultation-Liaison Psychiatry
Psychosomatics 35(3): p. 279 – 296, 1994

T.N. Wise, L.S. Mann, R. Silverstein & J. Steg
Consultation-Liaison Outcome Evaluation System (CLOES): Resident or Private Physicians' Concordance With Consultants' Recommendations
Comprehensive Psychiatry 28(5): p. 430 – 436, 1987

J. Zimmer
Length of Stay and Hospital Bed Misutilization
Medical Care 14: p. 453 – 462, 1974

Sigmundoscopy — The Bases

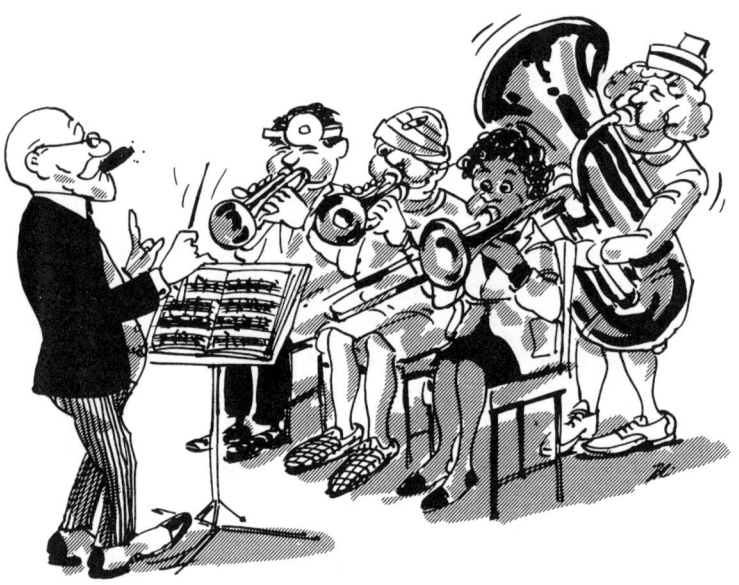

3/ Conducting the Consult

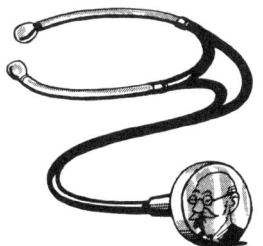

The next three chapters provide an overview on performing a psychiatric consultation, which involves the following steps:

- **The Referral**
- **Preparing for the Consult**
- **Interviewing the Patient**
- **Writing the Consultation Report** — discussed in the
- **Implementing the Treatment Plan** — following chapters

Consultation requests are initiated by phone, letter or personal contact. Keeping a central registry of medical and demographic information is frequently done and helpful for a variety of clinical, administrative and research purposes.

It is a common occurrence for other services to ask for an informal consultation (often called a "curbside"). This may be appropriate between consultants or in a non-teaching center, but has significant disadvantages for students and residents. The experience of performing a complete consult is lost, as is the opportunity of offering more to the patient than simply answering a clinical question or two. Each supervisor will have his or her own policy and rationale, but in general it is not good clinical practice to reduce a consultation to a single clinical point without the benefit of more information or interviewing the patient. For example, if you are asked, "Which antipsychotic has strong sedative properties?" it may become a medicolegal issue if you suggest chlorpromazine for a patient who has a pre-existing seizure disorder that you weren't told about at the time.

The Referral

Many centers have preprinted forms for recording both consult requests and the actual consultations. If some demographic information isn't provided initially, it can be added after the consult has been completed. Having as much data as possible beforehand increases the effectiveness of your preparation and interview.

The following mnemonic summarizes the essential information to record when a consult is requested:

"I'M SURE"

Identifying factors (name, age, gender, marital status, race, religion, occupation, etc.)

Medical problem(s)

Source of referral (referring physician and service)

Urgency (routine, urgent, emergency)

Reason for referral

Expectations of the consultee

The **identifying factors**, as in any medical document, help develop a picture of the patient. Each factor has its own clinical implications and helps tailor your preparation for the consult. These factors also give the practical advantage of helping to recognize the patient on a busy medical or surgical ward. You may well pass the person in the hallway or need to identify him or her in a room of several people.

An awareness of the patient's **medical problem** is valuable to know before the consult. This helps keep your general medical knowledge current. Also, discussing the medical situation is a good way of initiating a consult interview.

Conducting the Consult

Knowing the **source** of the referral also helps with particular aspects of the consult. Different services and referring physicians have expectations and idiosyncrasies that, once understood, make the process easier and more effective. Aspects such as the protocol for getting investigations and treatment suggestions approved or the degree of detail expected varies considerably between referring sources.

It is crucial to clarify the **urgency** of the consult. Most C-L services have a time frame for inpatient and outpatient assessments (e.g. twenty-four hours and three days respectively). It is a good practice to inform the consultee approximately when to expect your visit. Urgent consults often need to be seen the morning or afternoon in which they are requested. Emergencies are usually relayed from consultant to consultant. For such occasions, it is helpful to have the following available:

- a **crisis team** with physical and chemical restraints
- a knowledge of the laws in your area regarding involuntary committal, rights advice and medicolegal forms
- phone numbers for the police and hospital security
- familiarity with non-violent crisis intervention

In general, all consults should be seen as soon as possible. The referring source has come to a point where your expertise and input are necessary. Prompt attention will be appreciated and reciprocated when you request consults. Simply performing the consult can be of benefit to the patient and referring team. For example:

- conducting the consult tells the patient that his or her problems have been heard and acted upon; many medical and surgical units are so busy that they do not have the time to explore psychosocial problems
- your investigations may reveal added biological precipitants or perpetuating factors for the patient's illness
- in appropriate cases, transfer to the psychiatry unit puts the patient in a more suitable milieu and frees up a bed (for which you should expect enduring gratitude)

Sigmundoscopy — The Bases

Some unpleasant events can occur if the consult is delayed:

- the patient may be discharged or may die
- the physician may change his or her mind
- the patient may decline the consult
- the clinical condition can worsen

The crux of the consult is of course the **reason for referral**. This becomes "the question" that has to be answered at the end of the assessment. Page fifty-seven lists the most common reasons for which psychiatric consults are requested.

◆ What if no reason for referral is given?

Despite the integral role the consult question plays, it is surprising how often it is omitted from the request. This is perhaps the reason why "consults" are sometimes sarcastically referred to as "insults." The consultee has obviously come to a point where he or she requests help for a patient's psychiatric problem, but may have trouble expressing a clear reason for the referral.

Some psychiatrists refuse to see consults until all of the preliminary information is provided. This approach may be gratifying for the egos of such individuals, and may have merit in that these clinicians are somewhat more fully informed before seeing the patient. However, this approach fails to consider that a vague or absent "reason" often indicates that a greater degree of assistance is needed, and that the psychiatric problem may be of a more serious nature (Golinger, 1985). Additionally, it can force the consultee into putting "something" down on the request to impel such consultants to see the patient. Even with straightforward cases, the reason listed on the consult form may not ultimately be the area of greatest importance. This has been aptly described by Schiff & Pilot (1959), who stated that psychiatric consultations *. . . stem from the referring physician's concerns, of which the most cogent are frequently not stated.* Lipowski (1967) added that *. . . the request may bear little relevance to the real nature of the problem, and that the more diffuse and unclear the message, the more likely the consultee is in need of assistance.*

Conducting the Consult

Some primary physicians will refer patients because they are not well acquainted with psychiatric problems. In other situations, it may be that serious psychiatric illnesses engender confusion and anxiety among referring physicians. The tolerance for disturbing or disruptive behaviors may be fairly low on medical/surgical units, especially with problems such as:

- noncompliance with medications or procedures
- wandering, agitated or highly vocal patients
- suicidal thoughts or gestures
- expression of strong affects

Some physicians grudgingly make referrals (and some make none at all) because to them it is an admission of not being "omniscient and omnipotent." It can be further demoralizing to have to append consult requests before patients will be seen (perhaps to the point where no request is made). In spite of the ultimate quality of your assessment, these preliminary matters can have an overriding effect on the whole consult (even an excellent consult may not restore rapport with an irritated referring physician).

Psychiatrists are among the physicians least likely to make consult requests, and may well perform less of a work-up for referrals than other services. For example, a referral to a cardiologist for an "abnormal heart rhythm" will often suffice. Having to further specify the type of arrhythmia and provide a preliminary interpretation of an EKG is beyond the expectations of a psychiatric service. It is beneficial to keep this in mind for the referrals we receive. Consult requests sent to psychiatrists are in general at least as well documented as referrals between other specialties, and may in fact contain more information.

Keep in mind that a vaguely worded reason for referral may well mean the presence of a serious psychiatric illness, and that even a clearly stated one may not be accurate. It is more the responsibility of C-L psychiatry to effectively manage patients than it is to educate our colleagues, especially on how to make "proper" referrals. A number of articles have investigated the resistance shown by non-psychiatric physicians to requesting consults.

Sigmundoscopy — The Bases

While the comparative ranking of different reasons varies between authors, the factors described were relatively similar:

Patient-Related
• patient's reaction is expectable based on his or her illness
• relationship with the patient may be harmed by the referral
• don't wish to deal with the issues brought about by the consult
• poor past experience with a psychiatrist
• don't want to "lose" patient to another physician

Psychiatrist-Related
• don't have faith in psychiatry
• don't believe a psychiatrist would help this particular problem
• primary physician should be able to handle the problem
• poor access to a psychiatrist
• cost of consult is too high — a social worker or psychologist can perform the same service for less
• wish to avoid having potential deficits in management highlighted
• don't want to have deficits in knowledge made obvious
• psychiatrists infrequently keep physicians informed re: patients' progress
• psychiatrists are not visible enough in the medical community (e.g. on hospital committees)

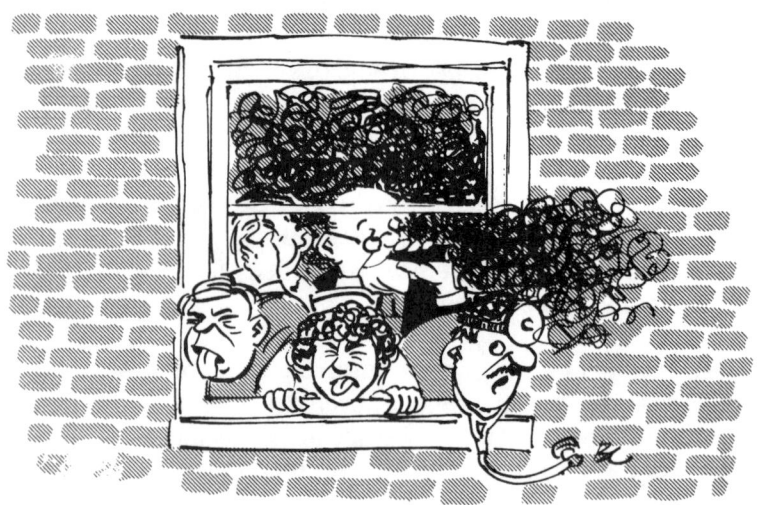

Who says we don't fit in?

Conducting the Consult

Along with the reason for the referral, the consultee often specifies **expectations** for the consult. Some centers include this as an additional check-box on consult forms. This is usually one of the following three possibilities:

- ❐ Please see and advise
- ❐ Please see and transfer care
- ❐ Please see and follow

The first option most commonly occurs in the following situations:

- starting, stopping or switching medications
- diagnostic clarification (including an opinion on whether or not a psychiatric illness is present)
- the patient is due to be discharged
- to arrange outpatient follow-up

The second option is usually requested in the following circumstances:

- patients who are "medically cleared" but have persisting psychiatric illnesses or ongoing suicidal ideation
- a locked unit or constant observation is needed for reasons of elopement or suicidal/homicidal ideation
- patients whose psychiatric illness poses more of a treatment concern than does the medical condition, and who can be managed medically if the referring source continues to follow the patient on the psychiatry unit

The most common arrangement involves a consult with follow-up visits provided for the duration of the admission. Even in cases where this isn't explicitly stated, continuing contact is appreciated and is good medical practice. The vast majority of studies reporting the benefits and positive impact of psychiatric consultations are based on assessments accompanied by ongoing visits. The usefulness of one-time only consultations is less clear, and intuitively this would seem to make a smaller impact because less time and effort has been devoted to determining the problem and helping the patient.

Sigmundoscopy — The Bases

Continuing to provide follow-up care has several advantages:

- additional history can be obtained from the patient
- assessing the day-to-day developments (e.g. Mini-Mental State Exam (**MMSE**) scores in a delirious patient)
- refining your diagnostic impression
- monitoring the effectiveness of your treatment suggestions and being able to adjust them as the need arises
- providing other consultation services beyond the one(s) requested (e.g. assessing financial competence)
- advising on the need or suitability of psychiatric care after discharge

Medical and surgical units are busy places. Rounds may be held early enough in the day that some patients are still asleep. Teaching seminars, procedures, new admissions, documentation, reading up on current cases and exam preparation all take time away from direct patient contact. Being in hospital becomes even more discouraging when people miss their doctors during rounds and wait for hours to get the chance to have their questions answered.

Staff on psychiatric consultation services often have the advantage of being able to spend longer periods of time with patients at flexible intervals. By seeing patients regularly, and at times other than morning or afternoon team rounds, we have the opportunity to become important figures in patients' treatment.

In using a "holistic" biopsychosocial approach, C-L service providers may well be the first or only ones to ask about certain aspects of patients' lives. All illnesses make an impact on patients' ability to function in social and occupational roles, which are areas our colleagues do not always have time to explore. We are also the most appropriate ones to assess the effectiveness of our treatment suggestions. For example, psychiatric C-L staff would be aware that antidepressants often treat the symptoms of depression in a predictable sequence and can document changes in mood, cognitive and vegetative signs instead of globally stating that someone "looks less depressed today."

Preparing for the Consult

Depending on factors such as level of training, supervisor's preferences, idiosyncrasies of the referring source, nature of the consult and knowledge of the medical problem, some preparation may be required before interviewing the patient. This process can be seen as an interaction between four entities:

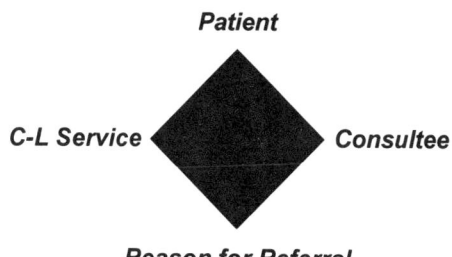

Each of these four factors contributes to the success of individual referrals and the ongoing usefulness of a C-L Service. If there isn't an understanding of, and balance between these factors, the consultation process can become unsatisfactory in any number of ways. For example:

1. The C-L resident makes an accurate diagnosis and initiates an effective treatment plan, but waited two days to see the patient when an urgent request was made.

2. The referring source neglects to authorize a suggested medication because a case report warns of the possibility of a (rare) complication. While the patient is willing to try the drug, the referring physician does not wish to take a calculated risk.

3. A consult is carried out in a timely fashion by an empathic, interested psychiatry resident. Several important issues are discovered which are fertile ground for psychotherapy. However, the resident doesn't know how to carry out the requested financial competence assessment.

4. In order to appease the C-L supervisor and the referring physician, a resident stays late to see a new referral. While the interview is complete, due to the hour, the resident is curt with the patient and takes shortcuts in writing the consult report.

Sigmundoscopy — The Bases

C-L Service expectations can and should be outlined at the beginning of a rotation. Experience with referring sources and dealing with a variety of problems provides the expertise for these aspects of the consult. Patient factors are always individual and can only be elucidated at the time of the consult.

While a cataloging of the possibilities in each of these four areas is beyond the scope of this book, the following are examples of selected factors:

◆ C-L Service Parameters

- Does the supervisor want to review all consults before they are seen? Only after they are seen? On a case-by-case basis?
- How quickly should consults be seen?
- How soon is the supervisor available to review new consults?
- Are there some treatments that can be started without direct supervision based on the residents' expertise? (e.g. antidepressant medication, bedtime sedation, etc.)
- What is expected in terms of documentation? (e.g. are notes to be written or dictated, length of notes)

◆ Consultee Parameters

- Can orders be written directly, or do they need to be cosigned by the C-L supervisor and/or physician?
- Is there an expectation for references (articles) to be provided with consults? (if so, how often and how many?)
- How likely is the consultee to implement suggestions? Does this vary for recommendations made for investigations, medications or psychotherapy?
- How much documentation does the referring source expect? Are the *impression* and *plan* parts all that matter?
- How interested is the consultee in learning about psychiatry? How much of an explanation for recommendations is required or desired?

Conducting the Consult

◆ Reason for Referral

• If another avenue becomes important to pursue, does the consultee have to give prior approval? (e.g. an initial request asks for sedation for a behaviorally disturbed patient, but the need arises to assess the person's capacity to consent to medical treatment)
• Should consultees who habitually provide scant documentation or unclear reasons for consultation be targeted for discussions to remedy this?

◆ Patient Parameters

• Was the patient informed of the consult?
• Did the patient request the consult? To what extent does the patient desire the consult?
• Has the person seen a psychiatrist or other mental health professional before?
• Is the patient currently capable of participating in an interview?

Touching base with a supervisor prior to the interview can be of practical assistance. The following examples illustrate how experience can help fine tune a consult.

• "Dr. Flannelette always gives blanket approval to our suggestions."

• "Dr. Gastrofreud likes to have her students sit in on the assessment — if the patient is agreeable."

• "Our inpatient ward is full at the moment, so don't make any commitments about a transfer to Dr. Turf."

• "That ward doesn't have an interview room, so call down to see if you can use the Hospital Administrator's private office."

• "Dr. Crunch only makes referrals at the last moment."

• "Speak to Dr. Nightingale's nurse before doing anything."

Sigmundoscopy — The Bases

◆ Chart Review

The following areas are of special significance in consultation psychiatry and need to be reviewed before seeing the patient.

Hospitalization Particulars
- length of hospital stay prior to the consult request?
- how did the patient come to medical attention?

Medical/Surgical History
- type, course and severity of the illness
- treatments currently being used and their efficacy
- plans for future investigations and treatment
- what has the patient been told about his or her condition and prognosis?

History of the Reasons for the Consultation
- precipitating and perpetuating factors
- exacerbations and remissions of behavioral problems
- possible association of changes in mental status with procedures, interventions, medications, etc.
- was anything brought in by visitors? (e.g. ethanol, pills from home, food, etc.)

Medication Review
- psychiatric complications of non-psychiatric medications (e.g. steroids, antihypertensives)
- pre-existing conditions made worse, or new medical problems caused by psychiatric medications

Laboratory Investigation Review
- has appropriate testing been carried out, and have the results been reported?
- have levels been drawn for applicable medications?
- is there an association between biochemical or hematologic abnormalities and altered mental status?

Review of Information
- check the emergency record and all multidisciplinary notes to obtain or corroborate information
- peruse old charts for relevant history

◆ Other Preparation

There are two other aspects that need to be attended to for the consult to occur smoothly and in a time-efficient manner.

Contact the Ward
With the increased emphasis on shortening the length of hospitalization, inpatient stays can involve one procedure after another. Calling ahead to ask about the patient's whereabouts and scheduling a time for the interview can prevent a wasted trip.

If the patient is off the floor, ask if a test is being done, and if so, where. This can help you gauge a time to return to the ward. Consults can also be performed in waiting areas (if suitable).

Patients may not speak English fluently, or even speak it at all. Interpreters can be arranged or family members can be asked to be present.

Brush up on the Medical/Surgical Problem
The patient's illness will have a large bearing on the consult. Your understanding of this illness is paramount to understanding the person and the difficulties he or she is experiencing.

Part of the subspecialty of C-L psychiatry involves knowing which illnesses and medications can precipitate or perpetuate changes in mental status. This requires a working knowledge (and frequent review) of physical medicine. This basis can also be helpful in the "detective work" of the consult. For example, in knowing that intravenous benzodiazepines are given for some procedures, you can make sense of an episode of disinhibited behavior.

One of the best ways of initiating a consult interview is to ask about the patient's illness, treatment, etc. Speaking knowledgeably about this establishes you as an expert and builds a common ground for you to then branch out into a more detailed psychiatric inquiry. Approaches to initiating the consult are provided later in this chapter.

Interviewing the Patient

Likely the most common obstacle in conducting consults is that the patient hasn't been informed of your visit. Mental illness still carries a stigma in society which unfortunately continues to extend to the hospital staff as well as the lay public.

This lack of notifying patients occurs so frequently that it has been the subject of a paper by Bagheri (1981). This study found that 68% of patients were not told that a psychiatric referral had been made. There was no correlation found between the rank or specialty of the referring physician and the likelihood of informing the patient.

The patient's medical/psychiatric problem seemed to have a bearing on the process of notification. Patients with personality or adjustment disorders were more likely to be told than those with psychotic disorders or organic brain syndromes.

Next, the authors asked referring physicians why they hadn't informed patients, and in a separate questionnaire, why they thought their colleagues might not do so. The results are as follows:

Reasons why referring physicians didn't inform patients (ranked from the most to the least common):

- didn't think of it
- too busy
- thought the patient wouldn't understand
- thought someone else had done it
- feared the patient may be offended

Reasons why physicians thought others making psychiatric referrals don't inform patients (from most to least common):

- patients would be insulted and become upset
- the consult may be refused by the patient
- it may damage rapport with referring physician
- the physician was too busy

Conducting the Consult

Omitting to inform patients about referrals is the end of a long chain of "challenges" faced by C-L psychiatry:

Many patients in general hospitals have psychiatric difficulties that are not detected by physicians.

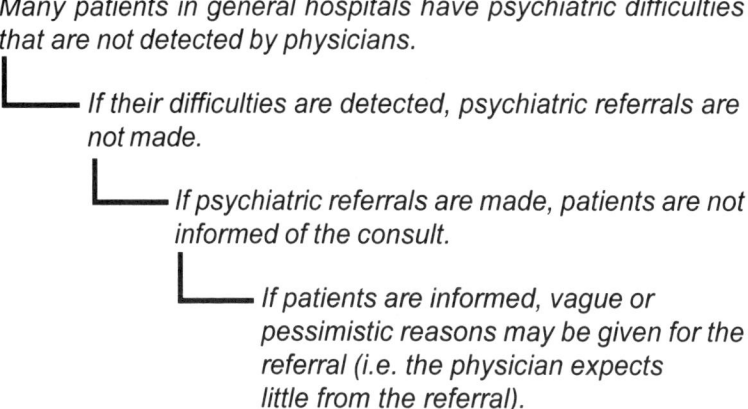

　— *If their difficulties are detected, psychiatric referrals are not made.*

　　— *If psychiatric referrals are made, patients are not informed of the consult.*

　　　— *If patients are informed, vague or pessimistic reasons may be given for the referral (i.e. the physician expects little from the referral).*

Referring physicians may choose not to inform patients about consults as a means of coping with their own ambivalence about the referral, or psychiatry in general. Another major factor is the fear of offending patients to the point of damaging rapport.

A study by Steinberg (1980) investigated the veracity of physicians' fears in not making referrals. Fifty patients, who had not originally been referred, had their charts reviewed regarding the suitability for a consultation. On this basis a consult was recommended, and agreed to, in twenty-nine cases. Of these, twenty-one were very receptive to the referral and five were deemed neutral. Wise (1985) found over 80% of patients accepted consults favorably. Despite physicians' reluctance, the great majority of patients view the intervention as positive.

It remains important to realize that a spectrum of attitudes towards psychiatry exists among our colleagues. Whether they are rationalizing their own reasons for not informing patients (e.g. too busy, someone else did it), or projecting their concerns onto patients (e.g. ruining rapport), it is a cogent point to keep in mind that many, if not the majority, of potential referrals aren't made.

◆ Approaches to Initiating the Consult

It is helpful to personally contact the referring source prior to the consult to obtain information for the following reasons:

- obtaining information not provided with the referral
- clarifying/verifying expectations
- getting a last-minute update on the patient's condition

As per the preceding section, you will be faced with speaking to patients who, in the majority of cases, don't know about the consult. You can use the pre-consult contact (meeting or phone call) with the referring source as an opportunity to ask if notification was given, and whether the physician will introduce you to the patient. This is ideal because it introduces the patient to a team/multidisciplinary approach to treatment. The introduction can benefit, rather than harm the relationship between the patient and the referring physician. Reluctant consultees can be told about the following benefits of a personal introduction:

- it indicates a mutual awareness that there is an emotional or psychiatric problem
- it demonstrates a willingness on the physician's part to arrange for the expertise needed to help
- it relieves primary physicians of having to deal with certain aspects of patients' care, and allows them to focus on their areas of expertise by identifying someone who will deal with these issues
- the clear majority of patients are receptive to psychiatric consultations

Some C-L psychiatrists expect that patients haven't been told about the referral and just see patients directly. Some will ask if an introduction can be made, but not insist on this. Others will not start the interview until the consultee accompanies them to see the patient. Again, while there is merit to each approach, it is important to keep in mind that referring physicians have reasons for not informing patients about visits from psychiatrists, and this too must be considered, and respected, in the overall consultation process.

Conducting the Consult

Ideally, an introduction to patients is made by the referring physician. Often this is brief, as shown by the following example:

> **Physician**: "Mr. XYY, we've spoken previously about your aggressive demeanor on this unit. I've asked one of my colleagues to speak with you to help out with this problem. This is Dr. Eager, he is a resident from the Department of Psychiatry."
> **Dr. Eager**: "Good morning, Mr. XYY. Are you feeling up to speaking with me right now?"
> **Mr. XYY**: "Absolutely, Dr. Eager."
> **Physician**: "Very well. I'll leave the two of you to talk."

More frequently, however, the C-L psychiatrist must independently inform patients that a consult has been requested. This engenders two difficulties, one being introducing the idea of the consult, and secondly that it is to occur at that moment.

In most cases, medical and surgical wards have rooms for one, two or four patients (usually called private, semi-private and quad/ward rooms respectively). While patients may, in general, be receptive to psychiatric consults, they are often less keen about their roommates knowing that one has been arranged.

Here are some suggestions for approaching this problem.

- have someone (usually the patient's nurse) take him or her to a private interview room
- introduce yourself as part of the medical or surgical team and ask if the patient would be agreeable to speaking in private where you can then give a fuller explanation
- speak in a hushed manner to preclude others from listening to your introduction
- ask the others in the room to step out for your interview (if this is reasonable and practical)
- introduce yourself as a psychiatric consultant and offer to conduct the interview elsewhere or at another time (which at least preserves confidentiality)

◆ Outline of the C-L Interview

The C-L interview has some unique qualities that set it apart from a general psychiatric interview.

For many patients, this is their first contact with a psychiatrist, or likely, any mental health professional. They usually have not been informed of your visit, may not agree with it, or see the rationale for why it was requested.

Patients won't know what is expected of them. They may only know about psychiatrists from their friends or the media. Jokes about mental illnesses are common, with references pervading many conversations. For example:

- "You've been acting kind of psychotic lately."
- "My supervisor has really lost his mind this time."
- "The voice in my head is telling me to take a vacation."

While the patient's friends and family may in the past have been teasing about his or her need to see a psychiatrist, finally meeting one is still another matter.

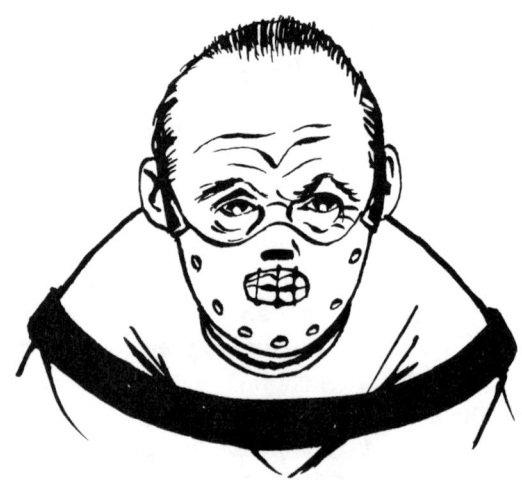

This may be what patients expect when they see you. And supposedly he was a good psychiatrist at one point!

Conducting the Consult

In contrast to some other types of psychiatric interviews, the C-L interview is usually quite active and engaging. An explanation detailing your position in the hospital and interest/expertise in psychiatry is frequently appropriate and helpful. A large number of people can be involved in patients' care on medical/surgical units. A detailed introduction is welcome, as is the opportunity to help patients match up the other names and faces to whom they have been exposed.

Keep in mind that the patient (usually) didn't request the consult — another doctor did. The onus is on you to develop rapport and facilitate the interview.

The following points are important to include at the beginning of the interview (though you can be flexible about the order):

- review the patient's medical problems and progress
- state the reason for the consult
- give an approximate idea of the length of the interview and broadly what you will be asking about
- you may need to obtain permission to speak with others (family members, family doctor, community psychiatrist, etc.) in order to obtain more information
- explain that you will have to provide a report (summary of the interview) back to the referring doctor, and you can't guarantee strict confidentiality of what the patient shares with you

In most cases, patients will speak quite readily, especially if you don't ask anything too "psychiatric" at the outset. Common approaches to focusing the interview are as follows:

- ask what the person's emotional reaction has been to the illness
- empathize with the degree of difficulty the person has had at work and in personal relationships
- indicate that the referring doctor was concerned, and ask in what way the person agrees with this opinion

Sigmundoscopy — The Bases

The priorities in conducting the consult interview are as follows:

1. Answer the consult question.

> This is essential. Keep this first and foremost in mind as you go through your preparation and interview. If the need arises, refine the request according to the situation.

2. Ask about other areas that will yield information relevant to the admission or management of the medical illness.

> Common areas that need exploration regardless of the consult request are: suicidal or homicidal ideation; capacity to consent to medical treatment (and in some cases capacity to manage finances); substance abuse.

3. Determine if the patient might benefit from ongoing psychiatric treatment (e.g. psychotherapy) for a condition that is not necessarily related to their medical illness.

> This can be part of a psychiatric "review of symptoms" that takes place if time permits. For example, an anxiety disorder discovered while asking a set of routine screening questions could be treated with cognitive therapy while the person is still in hospital.

Asking about the presence of other disorders can detect some of the rarer (or least reported) psychiatric conditions, such as: phobic disorders, delusional disorders, and some personality disorders, etc. However, trying to fulfil this third aspect can have potential drawbacks. Eliciting information not directly related to the consult question raises the issue of confidentiality. Should all information be put in a consult note? Should the consult note be placed on the medical chart where all disciplines have access to it? Should there be a brief note for the chart and a detailed one for the private records of the consultee? There is also the etiquette factor of not "stealing" patients. While you have a responsibility to the patient, situations that fall in this area should be cleared with, and arranged through, the referring physician.

Conducting the Consult

Consultation interviews tend to be short and focused. There are frequent interruptions, and often the patient cannot participate in a lengthy interview. This reinforces the need to prepare for the interview as completely as possible and to ask questions that yield the highest amount of information.

At times you may have to reword questions based on the presence of other patients or visitors in the room. There are certain areas that may have to be omitted because of their sensitivity (e.g. childhood sexual abuse) or because they have a lesser relevance to the consultation question (for example, some aspects of the personal and family history).

You will also have to tailor the interview to suit the nature of the request. A patient you are seeing only one time may require a more thorough interview than someone who will be in hospital for several weeks.

It is important to keep in mind that despite what the arrangement regarding admission appears to be at the time of the interview, this can and will change. Patients can be transferred to different hospitals, sign themselves out or be unexpectedly discharged. While there is always the opportunity to get more information in subsequent interviews, you may only be seeing the patient once, and for this reason, keep the consultation question in mind.

In a time-limited situation, it may be helpful to state the aim of your visit at the outset of the interview so you can redirect the patient to the salient matters if he or she heads off on a tangent. While most patients are cooperative and will speak with you readily, they do not usually know which pieces of information are essential and will need redirection at times.

Three other significant aspects of the C-L interview are:
- Splitting
- Regression
- The Mental Status Exam (MSE)

◆ Don't Split!

The process by which treatment or a "cure" comes about can vary considerably between psychiatry and medical/surgical units. Whereas psychiatric inpatients often receive direct attention daily from mental health professionals, physically ill patients are not always in need of this degree of interaction. Instead, medications and the body's ability to heal itself (time) are relied upon to a greater degree. For example, after surgery, a daily reassessment and fine-tuning of orders often provides good medical care.

When a psychiatric consultation is arranged, the patient may well have spent more time with you than he or she did with the referring doctor on that day, or even for several days. This, and being interested listeners, frequently puts consultants in the position of being a sounding board for patients' concerns. This occurs in three main contexts:

- complaints that the referring physician doesn't spend enough time with the patient, or doesn't spend as much time as you are able to
- comments to the effect that the physician doesn't explain procedures, discuss prognosis or tell the patient what to expect for the next step in the hospitalization
- telling you "secrets" that aren't to be shared with others

This process is called **splitting**, which is classified as a defense mechanism used by a person to deal with others whom are ambivalently regarded. The patient may come to regard you in the "all good" part of the split because you spend more time with him or her. Alternatively, you may become the "all bad" one because your presence indicates the person has a "mental disorder." Be vigilant for signs that splitting is occurring. Use this opportunity to defend the reputation of your colleagues and do not collude with an "us vs. them" attitude. If you have genuine concerns about someone's care, speak to the consultee directly. A common intervention in these situations is to have all the members of the treatment team (attending, nurses, housestaff, consultants, etc.) meet with the patient.

Conducting the Consult

◆ Regression

Regression refers to a decline in a patient's level of function, or the emergence of patterns from an earlier developmental stage. There are conscious and unconscious elements to this phenomenon. People regress in order to enjoy certain activities (sleep, sex, etc.), and the term **regression in service of the ego** describes situations (such as creativity) which are enhanced when fewer demands are imposed. Regression is also considered an **immature ego defense**, and as such, describes an attempt to avoid tension or conflict by returning (or falling back) to an earlier stage of personal development.

Regression occurs when people are under stress, and this happens to some extent in all inpatients. Previously high-functioning people, when afflicted by illness, will not be able to continue with their usual activities. Patients generally wear pajamas, spend the day in bed, sleep more than they do at home and have many of their responsibilities looked after by nursing staff. Additionally, patients are often in a recumbent position when they are seen. For these reasons, interview styles need to be adapted to consider the regression that occurs. For example, addressing patients by "Mr./Mrs./Ms." and asking them to sit up or take a chair (if possible) affords them a chance to preserve some of their dignity. Prefacing some of the parts of the MSE (i.e. cognitive functions) so they don't sound too basic for the patient is another means of addressing regression.

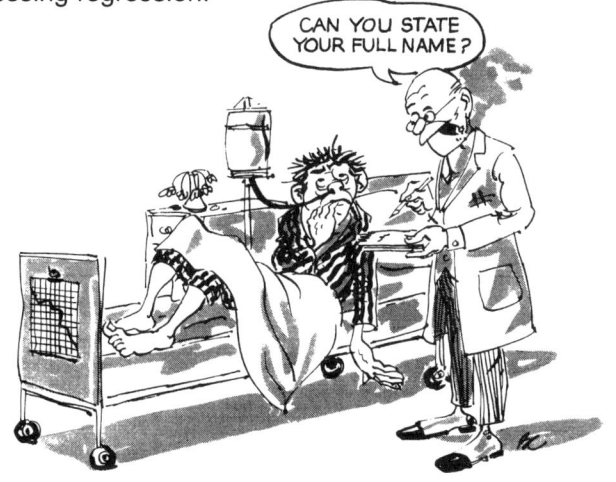

Sigmundoscopy — The Bases

◆ The Mental Status Exam (MSE)

The MSE is as critical to the psychiatric interview as the physical exam is to other areas of medicine. With cognitively impaired patients, such as those with delirium, advanced dementia or severe psychosis, the MSE may be the only part of the interview that is possible to perform.

The components of this exam are listed below. This mnemonic is helpful because it lists the parameters of the MSE in the order that they are often asked about and presented.

"ABC STAMP LICKER"*

Appearance
Behavior
Cooperation

Speech
Thought — **form** and **content**
Affect — visible moment to moment variation in emotion
Mood — subjective emotional tone throughout the interview
Perception — in all sensory modalities

Level of consciousness
Insight & Judgment
Cognitive functioning & Sensorium
        Orientation
        Memory
        Attention & Concentration
        Reading & Writing
Knowledge base
Endings — suicidal and/or homicidal ideation
Reliability of the information supplied

*From the book:
Brain Calipers
David J. Robinson, M.D.
© Rapid Psychler Press, 1997
ISBN 0-9680324-3-5, CD-ROM 0-9682094-0-8

Conducting the Consult

With time, C-L psychiatrists become very efficient interviewers and start the process of **hypothesis generation** soon after speaking to patients, and with a limited amount of information. The consultation interview differs from a standard psychiatric interview, an emergency room interview, and a psychotherapy assessment interview.

This is one of the few times when patients who (usually) did not request to see a psychiatrist are being asked to share personal information. C-L interviews frequently involve moving to a quiet room, asking others to give you privacy, speaking to patients while they are recumbent, etc. Discussions about medical problems and hospital issues commonly precede inquiries about areas in the psychiatric realm.

A warm, empathic greeting and thorough explanation is often required before information is gathered from the patient. The interviewer may need to work harder to gain rapport with patients in C-L interviews because of these factors.

The books below are recommended for gaining skills in psychiatric interviewing.

References for Interviewing Skills
Psychiatric Interviewing: The Art of Understanding, 2nd Ed.
S. Shea, M.D.
W.B. Saunders, Philadelphia, 1998

The Clinical Interview Using DSM-IV, Volume 1: The Fundamentals
E. Othmer, M.D., Ph.D & S. Othmer, Ph.D
American Psychiatric Press Inc., Washington D.C., 1994

The First Interview — Revised for DSM-IV
J. Morrison, M.D.
The Guilford Press, New York, 1994

Psychodynamic Psychiatry in Clinical Practice: The DSM-IV Ed.
G. Gabbard, M.D.
American Psychiatric Press Inc., Washington D.C.,1994

Interview Vignette

Dr. Eager: "Mr. Prazolam?"

Mr. Prazolam: "Yes."

Dr. Eager: "Good morning. I'm Dr. Eager, did Dr. Orthofreud say anything about my stopping by to speak with you?"

Mr. Prazolam: "Dr. Orthofreud . . . I haven't seen her since the operation two days ago. I'm glad you're here! I really want to get rid of this catheter. Oh, and while you're here, my usual medications haven't been given to me and I'm quite thirsty."

Dr. Eager: "Well, I'm here to help with some of those things, but I don't work on Dr. Orthofreud's team. I'm from the Psychiatry Department."

Mr. Prazolam: "That's just great. I break my hip, have an operation, lie here for two days not sleeping and now a shrink shows up. I suppose you're going to ask how I feel about that."

Dr. Eager: "How about if I explain a few things about what's happened, and then maybe you'll let me ask some questions."

Mr. Prazolam: "I'd sure like to know what's going on, but I'm not too happy about this."

Dr. Eager: "What in particular do you find upsetting?"

Mr. Prazolam: "Well, I broke my hip. I've had some pain and haven't slept well. Maybe I've been kind of nervous and edgy with the nurses. Now they send someone from your department."

Dr. Eager: "I can understand that you might be upset that no one told you I was coming to speak with you. Is there anything else about this that bothers you?"

Mr. Prazolam: "Yeah, sure. If they sent one of you people, it means everything I'm going through isn't real — it's all in my head, and now I'm cracking up. What's next? The men in white coats? A rubber room? I've seen *One Flew Over the Cuckoo's Nest*."

Conducting the Consult

Dr. Eager: "I saw the movie too. Frankly, if that was my only exposure to psychiatry, I'd be upset as well. Psychiatrists do a lot of different things, especially in general hospitals like this one."

Mr. Prazolam: "So why are you here?"

Dr. Eager: "As you mentioned a few minutes ago, I hear things haven't been going that well since the surgery. While you haven't seen Dr. Orthofreud, her team has been seeing you regularly and noticed the way things were going. They thought you seemed anxious, and at times, depressed. Also, they asked for advice on one of your medications. So you see, they have some pretty valid reasons for asking someone to speak with you."

Mr. Prazolam: "Well, wouldn't anyone be upset with a broken leg? You don't see everyone on this ward do you?"

Dr. Eager: "No, that's true. We only see people that we're specifically asked to see. Then we provide a report back to the attending physician, which in your case is Dr. Orthofreud."

Mr. Prazolam: "So what makes me so special?"

Dr. Eager: "I had a chance to read over your chart a couple of minutes ago so I have an idea what has happened. As far as I can understand — and please correct me if I'm wrong — it seems you were confused at home, became disoriented and fell down the stairs, causing you to break your hip."

Mr. Prazolam: "That's about right."

Dr. Eager: "Well, one of the medications you take is in the Valium® family, and it can sometimes cause people to become confused. There was some concern that you had taken some extra pills, and this might have led to the confusion."

Mr. Prazolam: "Yes, I did take some extras. They stopped calming my nerves, and I took more to just keep my head straight."

Dr. Eager: "Can you tell me what was going on before you increased the dosage? There's obviously some concern about you taking this medication again. Maybe another solution can be found."

Sigmundoscopy — The Bases

Mr. Prazolam: "This goes a few months back. You see, I was travelling down a highway and I noticed a car ahead of me start to weave in the lane. It was early in the morning so I didn't think it was a drunk driver and I followed for a couple of miles in case the driver pulled over with mechanical problems. Well, the guy had been up all night and fell asleep at the wheel. The car veered off the road and hit the concrete base of an overpass. I stopped as soon as I could, but the car immediately burst into flames and there was no way of getting close to the driver."

Dr. Eager: "That's terrible. What a shock it must have been."

Mr. Prazolam: "Yeah, it was terrible, alright. Anyway they figured the guy died on impact so it wasn't like he suffered or anything. But ever since then, I've had a lot of trouble focusing on my driving, especially when I'm on my own."

Dr. Eager: "What exactly is it that you experience?"

Mr. Prazolam: "I got these sudden flashes like my life was going to end — racing heart, trouble breathing, things like that."

Dr. Eager: "What did you do after this started happening?"

Mr. Prazolam: "I fought it for a while, then I went to see my family doctor and she started me on this medication. It worked pretty well for a while, but then it didn't do anything for me."

Dr. Eager: "Was that all that happened?"

Mr. Prazolam: "No, there was more. I kept feeling guilty about the guy. Here I was watching him bob around in the lane, maybe I should have beeped my horn or tried to get him to pull over."

Dr. Eager: "So there was some lingering guilt on your part as a result of the accident. How bad did this become?"

Mr. Prazolam: "I work as a truck driver. After the pills calmed me down, I was able to drive better but I couldn't focus as well. I started taking on more and more short runs, but they don't pay as good. Some of my expenses weren't being paid and I got pretty down about it because I'm usually paid right up."

Dr. Eager: "How would you say you were different than your usual self when you were feeling down?"

Mr. Prazolam: "I pretty much had trouble sleeping and concentrating on the job."

Dr. Eager: "Anything else?"

Mr. Prazolam: "That was it mainly. I started using more of those pills because I didn't feel as bad about my problems."

Dr. Eager: "How many were you taking when your use was at its highest?"

Mr. Prazolam: "At the most, it got to twenty pills a day."

Dr. Eager: "When did the fall occur?

Mr. Prazolam: "About four days after I starting taking that many."

Dr. Eager: "What else can you tell me about the days just before the fall?"

Mr. Prazolam: "Very little. It's really a blur to me now."

Dr. Eager: "Well, did things get so bad that you thought life wasn't worth living?"

Mr. Prazolam: "You mean like suicide? No, I didn't take them to overdose. Is that why you're here?"

Dr. Eager: "Partly for that, yes. I think you can understand how that would be something we'd ask about."

Mr. Prazolam: "Yeah, I guess so. But no, not me."

Dr. Eager: "I'm relieved to hear that, Mr. Prazolam. Another reason I'm here is to ask if you would be interested in a medication for your anxiety that didn't cause these sorts of problems, and in meeting someone on a regular basis to discuss what's happened to you? I think it would be helpful given all you've gone through."

Mr. Prazolam: "Sure. By the way, you can call me Al."

◆ The Consult as a Commodity

Many healthcare professionals eschew the application of business principles to their work. Nevertheless, a "commodity" analogy is a very cogent one for C-L psychiatry. As discussed, the interaction is far more extensive than a simple dyadic relationship between consultant and consultee.

Miller (1973) sought to define the consultation process more fully by using a **general systems model**. Guggenheim (1978), in an enjoyable and prophetic article, likened the model more to that of a marketplace where the consultation is seen as a product that must be effectively marketed.

An unfortunate reality in C-L psychiatry is that consult requests are optional for a significant percentage of patients. As discussed, process, local or even arbitrary variables are often the deciding factors as to whether referrals are made. Guggenheim aptly described this as being the major area where general systems theory fails to accurately define the consultation process:

Unfortunately, the theory as presented to date has not taken into account complexities of the general hospital as a sociological structure with powerful opinion-swinging constituencies that can accept or reject the consultant. It has also failed to focus on the consultant's roles as good will ambassador and salesman (in addition to his usual roles as physician, psychiatrist, and psychotherapist).

One's success in C-L psychiatry will certainly be influenced by the same factors that affect goods or services in the business world. One of the most important shifts in conceptualizing consult services in general hospitals is switching from a sales perspective ("This department has an excellent C-L service, how are you going to use it.") to a marketing perspective ("Tell us what you need from a C-L service and we will develop/deliver it."). Unfortunately, the ability to perform a consult fulfills only part of what is required. Burket (1993) found that the features most valued by pediatricians requesting psychiatric referrals were accessibility and a timely response from consultants. Just as in business, the C-L team's image and reputation will influence referral patterns.

Conducting the Consult

Accordingly, there are "marketplace" aspects to consultations:

> • **advertising** (e.g. letting consultees know about the progress/improvement of patients from past referrals)
> • **promotion** (e.g. your presence on the medical-surgical wards or at their rounds)
> • **merchandising** (e.g. tailoring aspects of the consultation (notes, recommendations, disposition, etc.) to suit consultees)

Because local variables (e.g. Dr. Froyd gets a lot of consults from Dr. Woods because they play golf together) so strongly influence the consultation process, it is helpful to see referring sources as customers on whom we rely for repeat business.

References for Consults as Commodities
W.B. Miller
Psychiatric Consultation I: A General Systems Approach
Psychiatric Medicine 4: p. 135 — 146, 1973

F.G. Guggenheim
A Marketplace Model of Consultation Psychiatry in the General Hospital
American Journal of Psychiatry 135(11): p. 1380 — 1383, 1978

R.C. Burket & J.D. Hodgin
Pediatricians' Perceptions of Child Psychiatry Consultations
Psychosomatics 34(5): p. 402 — 408, 1993

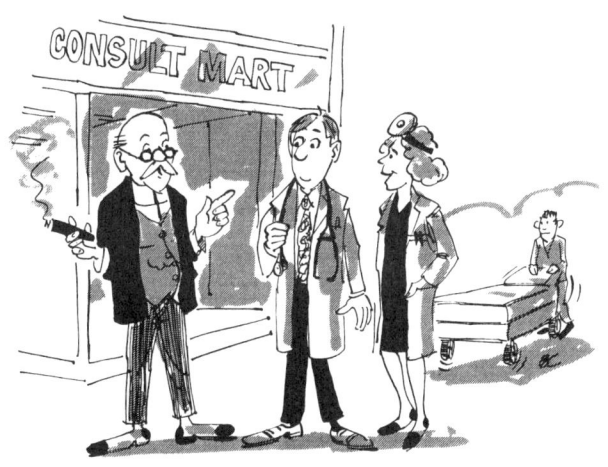

Sigmundoscopy — The Bases

Summary
Psychiatric consultations, like all medical interventions, require proper planning and an understanding of the interplay of the integral factors:

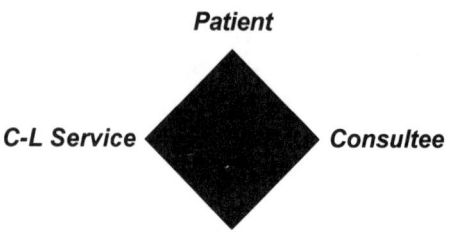

Patient

C-L Service   *Consultee*

Reason for Referral

◆ **The Referral**
  • get all the information you can when the consult is requested — remember the mnemonic, **"I'M SURE"**
  • determine *the question* the consultee is asking, and what kind of intervention is being requested

◆ **Preparing for the Consult**
  • review the basics of the medical/surgical problem
  • read all available information (medical chart, old charts, letters, etc.)
  • call the ward to find out about the patient's availability, ability to speak English, etc. and to arrange a time and room
  • speak to the referring source for last minute information concerning the consult, ask if the patient was informed of the consult and arrange a personal introduction

◆ **Interviewing the Patient**
  • conduct the consult as soon as possible
  • spend time developing rapport with the patient before shifting to matters of psychiatric relevance
  • inform the patient of the purpose of the interview and that a written note will be sent back to the referring doctor
  • obtain written consent to speak with others (family, G.P., government agencies, other hospitals, etc.)
  • first and foremost answer the consult question
  • perform a complete mental status examination

References

A.S. Bagheri, L.S. Lane, F.M. Kline & D.M. Araujo
Why Physicians Fail to Tell Patients A Psychiatrist Is Coming
Psychosomatics 22(5): p. 407 — 419, 1981

P.J. Fink
Dealing With Psychiatry's Stigma
Hospital & Community Psychiatry 37: p. 814 — 818, 1987

R. Golinger, M.L. Teitelbaum & M.F. Folstein
Clarity of Request for Consultation: Its Relationship to Psychiatric Diagnosis
Psychosomatics 26(8): p. 649 — 653, 1985

Z.J. Lipowski
Review of Consultation Psychiatry and Psychosomatic Medicine
Psychosomatic Medicine 29: p. 153 — 171, 1967

Z. J. Lipowski
Consultation-Liaison Psychiatry: An Overview
American Journal of Psychiatry 131: p. 623 — 630, 1974

S.K. Schiff & M.L. Pilot
An Approach to Psychiatric Consultation in a General Hospital
Archives of General Psychiatry 1: p. 349 — 357, 1959

H. Steinberg, M. Torem & S.M. Saravary
An Analysis of Physician Resistance to Psychiatric Consultation
Archives of General Psychiatry 37: p. 1007 — 1012, 1980

T.L. Thompson II, T.N. Wise, A.B. Kelley & L.S. Mann
Improving Psychiatric Consultations to Nonpsychiatric Physicians
Psychosomatics 31(1), p. 80 — 84, 1990

J. Wallen, H.A. Pincus, H. H. Goldman & S.E. Markus
Psychiatric Consultation in Short-term General Hospitals
Archives of General Psychiatry 44:p. 163 — 168, 1987

T.N. Wise
What to Expect From a Psychiatric Consultant
Primary Care 4: p. 661— 668, 1977

T.N. Wise, L.S. Manley, H.W. Dove, E. Pluchik & K.W. Keirnan
Patients' Perceptions of Psychiatric Consultations
Comprehensive Psychiatry 26(6): p. 554 — 557, 1985

Sigmundoscopy — The Bases

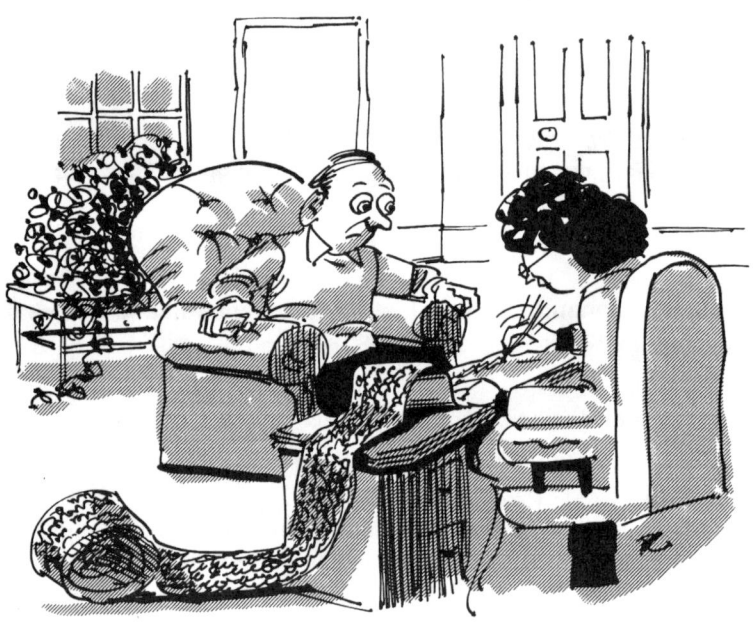

The Consult Report & Recommendations

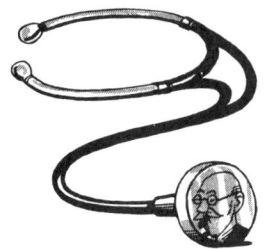

4/ The Consultation Report

The consultation report is a unique medical document. It differs from other notes by not being written primarily for medico-legal reasons, to record progress or assist the writer's memory. The consult note serves several, and at times contradictory, functions.

In Theory ☺	In Reality ☹
The note is a doctor-to-doctor communication...	The consult may have been initiated by the patient, family, etc.
The note should be thorough...	Interest in the note is often inversely proportional to its length
Medical records should be kept confidential...	The note is placed on the chart for all clinical services to see — including reviews for research and insurance purposes
The note contains an outline for a treatment plan...	Recommendations do not automatically become orders because the patient is not under the direct care of the consultant
The note should be an accurate record of the interview...	Patients can review their records at any time and may see certain aspects as pejorative (such as descriptions of their appearance or behavior, or when certain diagnoses are given)

Goals for the Consultation Report

- above all else, answer the consult question
- succinctly summarize the psychiatric problems; Popkin (1980) found that with a shorter note, there was a higher chance that drug recommendations were implemented
- include a *Review of Symptoms* and *Mental Status Exam* to document the rationale for how you formed your diagnostic impression and treatment plan
- outline a practical treatment plan involving biological, social and psychological factors with appropriate investigations and short/longer term treatments
- if desired and appropriate, provide a brief, focused educational aspect to the consult (which can include actual articles, references and personal experiences)

Many clinicians take notes during the interview, especially to record the cognitive functions in the MSE. These notes are useful to refer to when composing a formal consultation report but are unlikely to be sufficient in their original form.

It is a common practice to include a handwritten note, usually from one to three pages in length, at the end of the consult. This provides immediate feedback for the consultee. Another popular practice is to speak with the referring source after the consult, often to give your opinion and present treatment options. This discussion can include the highlights of your findings, but rarely includes all the detail that would be contained in a consult note.

Depending on service requirements and the availability of clerical staff, a second dictated note is also sometimes provided. This note is usually more detailed, and can serve as a record for findings or impressions that are tactfully left off the chart on the medical floor. Notes of this type are especially helpful for patients:

- with complicated histories
- with sensitive historical information
- who are likely to require repeat (future) consultations

The Consult Report & Recommendations

Despite the many advantages of speaking with referring sources both before and after the consult, your note may be the only contact they have with the C-L Service. If your sole interaction with others is going to take place via the chart, then your initial note becomes the calling card which sets the stage for the nature and quality of further exchanges. Future perusers of the medical chart will attest to your brilliance (or otherwise) based on your ability to compose a crisp, accurate and useful note.

For this reason, it is useful to consider your note as being an ambassador to the foreign territory of medical-surgical units. This concept will be expanded further in outlining the sections generally included in a consult note.

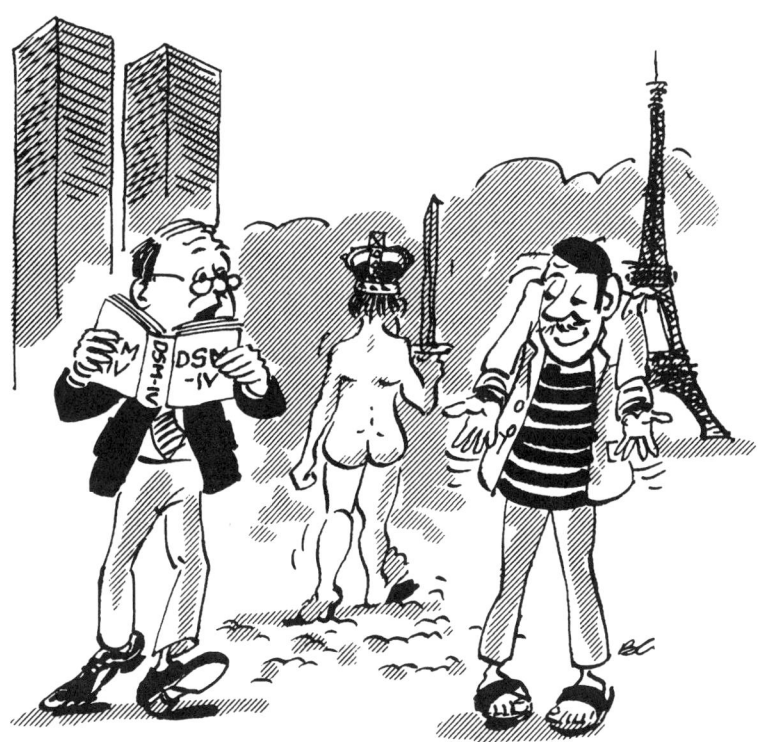

Don't just dispatch a Page, send an Ambassador!

The Well-Composed Ambassador
A well-written consultation note blends art and science. Here are the key elements for composing your psychiatric ambassador:

◆ *A Sense of Entitlement*
The consultation note requires a title. Some departments have preprinted forms with a prominent heading, as well as check boxes for other relevant information. Most hospitals have generic consult forms for all services. These frequently come assembled as carbonless copies so that the referring physician, medical records and the consultant can all have a copy. Lastly, if no forms are available, the note can be written on hospital paper and placed in the "Consultations" or "Progress" section of the chart.

◆ *A Proper Introduction*
A one or two sentence "identifying statement" usually starts off the formal note. These parameters are often relevant to the prognosis and treatment planning, and are important to include at the outset. However, the referring source already knows this information, so be brief. It is vital to include the date of the interview, often with the time (and time period) the person was seen. Some clinicians routinely list the sources of information used in the consult (e.g. patient, family, general practitioner, chart, etc.). Others only include this information if the assessment is incomplete, or if the patient was not the primary source of data. The length of stay in hospital prior to the consult can also be included.

◆ *A Well-Informed Opening*
After the identifying information, it is common to include a one or two sentence summary of the patient's:

- medical or surgical problem/reason for admission
- course and severity
- recent or proposed procedures

Again, this information is known to the referring source. Brevity is advisable because you haven't as yet added anything new — so include only what is relevant to the immediate problem.

The Consult Report & Recommendations

◆ A Clear Sense of Purpose
The next section states the reason for the referral and possibly the consultee's expectations. This can consist of simply restating the request, rewording it into a more typical request, or in cases where the reason wasn't explicitly stated, describing what to you seems to be the most appropriate reason for the referral. As stated previously, the reason for referral is often omitted from the consult request, but is important to include in a formal note.

This is also not the time or place to involve sarcasm or highlighting the lack of psychological mindedness of some of our colleagues. Requests such as the following should be reworded:
- "Please stop this patient's hallucinations"
- "Assess and change the patient's personality"
- "Tell the patient to be nicer to the nursing staff"
- "Advise on proper anticonfusional medication"

The reason for referral becomes the focus of the consult. Along with an understanding of the consultee's expectations, this forms the basis of your recommended treatment plan, and in a sense forms the "contract" for the consult.

◆ A Thorough Grounding in Current Events
The next section, the **History of Presenting Illness (HPI)**, details the events leading up to the consult request. This section starts at the point where the patient was last well (or was last his or her "usual self") and details the medical, psychiatric and interpersonal factors necessary to understand how the person came to be in the current situation at the time the consult was requested.

This section diverges from the medical/surgical style and takes on a distinctly psychiatric flavor. Symptoms are presented which are relevant to the medical problem and which lead to a psychiatric diagnosis. All aspects which are relevant to the patient's current difficulties are listed here. These can include factors such as medications, family and job stresses, substance abuse, etc. Significant negative findings are also listed in this section.

Sigmundoscopy — The Bases

◆ Understanding Past as Prologue

The **psychiatric history** is often the next section included, which chronicles the following information:

- previous admissions
- other contact with mental health professionals
- type, duration and response to psychotherapy
- treatment with medications and outcome
- substance abuse that is in remission or considered not contributing to the current difficulties

For the sake of brevity, this section can also be used for recording information that might be placed in the Personal/Social and Family History in a full psychiatric history. Other significant aspects that can be recorded in this section are:

- previous losses
- past responses to stressful events
- characteristic coping patterns (personality style)
- anniversary dates of significant losses
- relatives affected by psychiatric conditions

◆ The Directive of the "Mental State"

The **MSE** is an essential area of evaluation in consultation psychiatry. This structured set of inquiries assesses cognitive functions and the symptoms of psychiatric illness not covered elsewhere in the interview. Documenting the MSE is like recording the "objective" part of the **S.O.A.P.** assessment. Positive findings from the MSE illustrate how psychiatric diagnoses and recommendations are based on detailed, structured inquiries.

The MSE has a significant likelihood of being abnormal because of the higher prevalence of cognitive impairment (delirium, dementia, etc.) in medically ill patients with psychiatric problems. Remember that the MSE is a snapshot of a person's mental functioning — it can and will vary with time. The MSE can be supplemented with other cognitive screening tests like the **Mini-Mental State Exam (MMSE)** and clock drawing.

The Consult Report & Recommendations

◆ Seeing Between The Lines

A **Review of Symptoms (ROS)** is frequently included in consultation notes. For many patients who are referred, the consult will be their only contact with a psychiatrist. Exploring other diagnostic possibilities which are related to the core symptoms is a very worthwhile exercise because:

- it helps detect occult psychiatric illnesses
- it establishes you as a thorough consultant, and the referring source will (hopefully) request more consults

While the questions in this area can take a few minutes to ask, the documentation can be brief. You can list the individual psychiatric conditions screened for as being not present, or list the overall categories. For example:

- "Negative screen for psychotic, anxiety and somatoform disorders"
- "Screened for anxiety disorders other than Panic Disorder — OCD, PTSD, Phobias (including Agoraphobia) & GAD not present"

◆ A Unifying Stance

An **impression**, **summary** or **formulation** follows next. Many times, this and the proposed treatment plan will be all that the primary physician reads. This section is usually a paragraph in length and starts with significant identifying factors and the medical problem and course/severity of that illness.

Then, the positive psychiatric symptoms are highlighted and correlated into a **provisional**, **preferred** or **working diagnosis**. A **differential diagnosis** is also included, and may be emphasized in cases with higher degrees of complexity. Detailing the process of collecting information from the patient (and other sources), identifying symptoms and then distilling them into a diagnostic formulation makes your rationale for suggesting investigations and treatments (both biological or psychosocial) clear to the referring source and increases the likelihood of their implementation.

◆ Treatment Planning & Recommendations

If the previous sections of the consult note answer the question, *"What is going on with this patient?"* then the treatment plan answers the question, *"What do we do about it?"* Primary physicians have a varying interest in your ability to conduct an interview and arrive at an elegant diagnostic formulation, but there will be universal interest in your expertise in directly helping to manage their patients. Your treatment plan is the most important part of the consult and may be the only part that gets read. Generally, your outline becomes a list of suggestions for the referring team and they may or may not agree with your ideas. The degree to which consultees follow recommendations has been termed **concordance**, and is discussed in a separate chapter.

Following a biopsychosocial outline, one approach is to consider which investigations are called for, and then which short and longer-term treatments will benefit the patient. An outline of the most common parameters in these areas appears in the next section.

Investigations are most frequently ordered to help distinguish disorders that have a demonstrable physiologic basis. Such disorders are still frequently called "organic," to draw a distinction from causes deemed to be entirely psychiatric or "functional" illnesses (sometimes still called "supratentorial"). The DSM-IV terminology for this is **Mental Disorder Due to a General Medical Condition**. For example, someone who clearly develops a major depressive episode due to Cushing's Disease would be diagnosed in the following manner:

Axis I   Mood Disorder due to Cushing's Disease, with Depressive Features
Axis III Cushing's Disease

Where the etiology is less clearly related, the diagnosis would be recorded as:

Axis I   Major Depressive Disorder
Axis III Cushing's Disease

The Consult Report & Recommendations

Biopsychosocial Management Plan

> **Assessment in a clinic or outpatient setting**
> - Is admission to hospital necessary?
> - Does the patient warrant an involuntary admission?

Investigations

Biological
- Admission physical exam
- Diagnostic tests:
    Routine: hematologic and clinical chemistry admission/screening bloodwork
    Toxicology: serum medication levels; urine screen for substances of abuse
    Special assays
- Diagnostic investigations: CXR, EKG
- Neuroimaging: CT, MRI scans
- EEG
- Consultations to other medical/surgical specialties
- Special tests:
    hypothalamic/pituitary/adrenal axis testing (DST, TRH stimulation test, GH response)
    sleep studies
    other

Social
- Collateral history:
    friends and family members
    primary care physician
    community psychiatrist
    other clinics, programs or hospitals
- Activities of Daily Living (**ADL**) assessment
- Referral to members of multidisciplinary team
    social worker
    occupational therapist
    physiotherapist
    dietician
    clergy
    nurse clinician

Psychological
- Personality and Intelligence tests
- Cognitive screening tests (e.g. Mini-Mental State Exam, Clock Drawing, etc.)
- Neuropsychological test batteries
- Structured interviews/diagnostic testing

Sigmundoscopy — The Bases

Treatment — Short Term

Biological
- Psychopharmacology
    - *antidepressants*
    - *antiparkinsonian agents*
    - *antipsychotics*
    - *anxiolytics*
    - *mood stabilizers*
    - *psychostimulants*
    - *sedative/hypnotics*
    - *other*
- ECT
- Other psychiatric treatments
- Somatic illnesses
    - *medications*
    - *physical treatments*
- Detoxification from medications or substances
- Environmental
    - *level of observation*
    - *passes*
    - *attire (pajamas or street clothes)*
    - *seclusion rooms*
    - *mechanical restraints*
    - *objects to assist with reorientation*

Social
- Social services
    - *assistance with housing, finances, etc.*
- Education and focus/support groups
- Occupational Therapy
- Family meetings
- Administrative
    - *voluntary/involuntary status*
    - *rights/legal advice*
    - *duty to warn/duty to protect others*
    - *treatment contracts*
    - *informing work/school of absence*
    - *substitute consent if deemed incapable*

Psychological
- Advice/Reality Therapy
- Behavior Therapy/Modification
- Cognitive Therapy
- Group Therapy
- Milieu Therapy
- Recreation Therapy
- Stress Management/Coping Skills
- Other therapies with a shorter-term focus

The Consult Report & Recommendations

Treatment — Longer Term

Biological
- Reduction/optimization of dosage
- Depot antipsychotic medications
- Monitoring vulnerable organ systems
- Serum level monitoring
- Adjunct/augmentation/combination treatments
- Factors reducing the efficacy of medication
  - *nicotine*
  - *caffeine*
  - *liver enzyme inducers*
  - *others*
- Health teaching and lifestyle changes

Social
- Vocational rehabilitation
- Religious guidance
- Community supports and organizations
- Discharge planning
  - *transfer to another facility*
  - *housing options*
  - *case manager*
- Liaison with general practitioner

Psychological
- Psychotherapy
  - *continuation of inpatient therapy*
  - *arrange outpatient treatment*
- Match various types of therapies to needs and attainable goals for the patient
- Types of therapies listed two pages ahead

The Biopsychosocial Grid *

	Biological	Psychological	Social
Investigations	A	B	B
Short-Term Treatment	C	E	F
Longer-Term Treatment	D	E	F

* the letters refer to the sections on the following pages where these topics are discussed in detail

Sigmundoscopy — The Bases

◆ Medical Differential Diagnosis

"MASTER THIS SCID"*

Metabolic
Autoimmune
Septic/Infectious
Traumatic
Endocrine
Renal

> SCID stands for the Structured Clinical Interview for the DSM-IV

Toxic
Hematologic/Circulatory
Idiopathic
Structural

Somatoform (Psychiatric)
Congenital
Iatrogenic
Degenerative

"VITAMIN CDE"*

Vascular
Infectious
Traumatic
Autoimmune
Metabolic
Idiopathic
Neoplasm

Congenital
Drug Induced (Iatrogenic)
Endocrine

The Consult Report & Recommendations

◆ Treatment Modalities

"ABCDEFGHIJKLMN"*

Addiction
Behavioral
Cognitive
Drug (medications)
ECT (electroconvulsive therapy)
Family Therapy
Group Therapy
Hospitalization (partial, day or inpatient)
Insight-Oriented (psychoanalysis, psychodynamic psychotherapy)
Job (vocational rehabilitation)
Knowledge (patient and family education)
Leisure (art therapy, music therapy, crafts groups, etc.)
Marital and relationship counseling
Novel treatments (even psychoanalysis was a fad at one time!)

*From the book:
Psychiatric Mnemonics & Clinical Guides, Second Edition
David J. Robinson, M.D.
© Rapid Psychler Press, 1998
ISBN 0-9682094-1-6

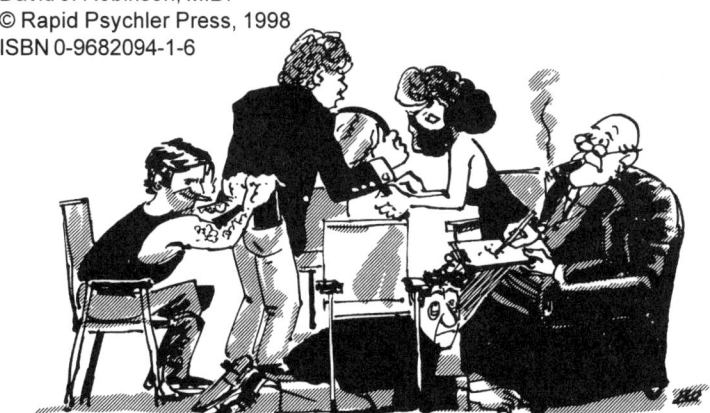

A/ Biological Investigations

Recommending biological investigations can at times be a delicate issue. Most referrals will come to you from experts in physical medicine who will at least have initiated investigations (being "worked-up"), if not having already ordered thorough testing for their patients. With the costs of medical care escalating, many physicians are being conservative in which tests are ordered (i.e. serum levels of ozone, porcelain and marmalade are no longer routine). For this reason, certain investigations may have been considered and postponed pending clinical necessity (i.e. waiting for more common tests to be reported as within normal limits (WNL) before investigating less common possibilities).

Your suggestions may not be implemented because they are thought to be a low-yield proposition. Referring physicians generally do not look for psychiatric consults to direct them to order more investigations, since this is their area of expertise. Keep in mind that requesting consultations can be difficult for physicians because in asking for assistance, it is a reminder that they are not "all capable and all knowing." While many physicians accept that psychiatry is different enough from physical medicine that they will readily request your help, recommendations for biochemical or hematologic tests may be misconstrued to mean that you don't feel they are demonstrating capable medical skills.

Explaining the clinical necessity of your ideas rather than exchanging notes in the chart goes a long way to insuring that they will be carried out. If you have a high index of suspicion, work collaboratively with the referring team by telling them your concerns and allowing them to direct the investigations.

The tests most likely to be accepted are those that fall under the domain of psychiatry. For example, the ordering of lithium, carbamazepine or valproate levels is often not done routinely and will be relevant to the consult. Additionally, testing of organ systems affected by such medications (e.g. liver function tests, blood cell counts, thyroid function) is more likely to be carried out.

The Consult Report & Recommendations

Alternatively, not every member of every team considers the myriad of psychological consequences that can be caused or maintained by physical illnesses.

There are certain situations that may require you to order routine tests or to be more assertive in seeing that your suggestions are carried out:

- *Beginning of rotations or academic years.*
- *Temporary lack of supervision for a medical team.*
    Medical students, clinical clerks, residents, fellows and students in other clinical programs work in hospitals because an apprenticeship is required in addition to classroom material. No one learns to swim by reading a book, and this is reflected in the often heard statement, "the last time I saw a textbook case was in a textbook." Junior housestaff may, at times, need a hand to learn how to manage cases. Since there is an overlap between all medical fields, your experience may be of assistance beyond the usual role of a consultant.
- *Referral early in the admission.*
    Some consults are requested at the outset of an admission and not all the tests will have been ordered prior to your visit. While it is always a benefit to being called earlier than later, you may need to postpone your investigations or recommendations pending the test results.

In the vast majority of cases, adequate testing will have been ordered. However, you may find that not all results have been reported and you can call the lab for the values.

You may infrequently discover a medical disorder that hasn't yet been detected (e.g. Wilson's Disease, lead poisoning, hypothyroidism). In general, consultees appear more interested in management recommendations than in investigations (Popkin, 1983). However, Popkin (1982) also found that consultees have an inclination to prematurely terminate the work-up of patients with psychiatric symptoms.

Sigmundoscopy — The Bases

◆ **Important Organic Considerations**

"TIME WON'T PASS"

Trauma — particularly head injuries and intracranial bleeding
Infections — especially of the CNS
Multiple sclerosis
Epilepsy

Wilson's Disease — an inherited defect in copper metabolism
Obstruction of CSF — Normal Pressure Hydrocephalus (NPH)
Nutritional — e.g. vitamin deficiencies, protein-deficient diets
Toxic — ingestion of medication, heavy metals, chemicals, etc.

Porphyria, **P**heochromocytoma
Axis of hypothalamus-pituitary-thyroid-adrenal glands
Space-Occupying Lesions
Substances — abuse, tolerance, intoxication and withdrawal states

Hall (1980) investigated the prevalence of medical illnesses that caused or exacerbated psychiatric symptoms (left column below). The right column lists the investigations useful in detecting these illnesses. These investigations are ranked by Hall from most to least useful:

Illnesses
- Endocrine   43%
- CNS   19%
- Hematologic   19%
- Cardiovascular   9%
- Gastrointestinal   6%
- Genitourinary   2%
- Musculoskeletal   2%

Investigations
- Blood chemistry — 34 panel
- Complete physical exam
- History
- Complete blood count
- Blood chemistry — 12 panel
- Sleep-deprived EEG
- ECG
- Routine urinalysis
- Cursory physical exam
- Complete neurological exam

B/ Social & Psychological Investigations

These investigations are far less likely to rankle consultees. Such investigations traditionally fall under the rubric of the behavioral sciences and are not typically assessments that the referring team would or could carry out without your help.

In the interest of efficiency, check to see if anyone from the referring team has undertaken any of the following actions:

- requested old charts
- contacted the family doctor
- arranged a family meeting

Usually you will be required to speak with the collateral sources of information that are more socially/psychologically oriented. This usually involves contacting: mental health professionals, community agencies, schools or places of employment. Pharmacies are also important sources of information.

On occasion, specialized neuropsychological testing will be necessary (the deficits to be further explored will of course be detected in your initial MSE). The most common mental functions assessed are: memory; reasoning and problem solving; perceptual performance; intelligence; language; motor skills; orientation, attention & concentration. Some of the tests most frequently ordered to assess mental functions are:

- Luria-Nebraska Neuropsychologic Battery
- Halsted-Reitan Battery
- Wisconsin Card Sorting Test
- Wechsler Adult Intelligence Scale — Revised (**WAIS-R**)
- Assessment of Daily Living (**ADL**s)

Other psychological testing may be needed to assess personality. These are divided into **objective tests** (e.g. MMPI) and **projective tests** (e.g. Rorschach, Thematic Appercertion Test, etc.). In order to more fully document your diagnoses, there are various Structured Clinical Diagnostic Assessments.

C/ Short-Term Biological (Psychopharmacological) Treatments

Having a facility with the indications, side-effects and contraindications of both psychiatric and non-psychiatric medications is a necessity in C-L psychiatry. Psychiatric drugs can cause a wide variety of medical complications (e.g. orthostatic hypotension, hepatotoxicity, galactorrhea/amenorrhea, agranulocytosis, etc.). Similarly, drugs for medical conditions can cause a plethora of psychological reactions (mania, depression, psychosis, anxiety, dissociation, sleep disorders, personality changes, etc.). While the list of possible reactions is quite extensive, it is imperative to keep the more common sequelae in mind. An important clinical pearl in this regard is to always keep an index of suspicion and look for factors that may have precipitated the patient's difficulties.

Because of the decreasing length of inpatient stays, medications are a very important part of a consultant's armamentarium. Many agents will work in a span of hours to days (e.g. benzodiazepines, antipsychotics). While some have a longer period to onset (e.g. mood stabilizers, antidepressants), it is important to get such medications started as soon as possible.

A question to always consider is, "At this time, what is/are the right psychiatric medication(s) for a patient with these physical illnesses?" Dealing with inpatients holds advantages in the area of psychopharmacology:

- compliance is very good (but not 100%)
- a variety of routes of administration are possible (oral, intravenous, sublingual, rectal, intramuscular, transdermal)
- you have the chance to monitor daily progress
- there are many caregivers to assess side effects
- serious reactions/side effects can be dealt with quickly

On the other hand, inpatient prescribing does have special concerns. Patients may be cognitively impaired and not be able to give informed consent. There may be factors related to hospitalization (noisy rooms, bad food) that get reported as side effects (poor sleep and decreased appetite, respectively).

The Consult Report & Recommendations

While a comprehensive discussion of C-L psychopharmacology is beyond the scope of this book, a list of some of the more relevant clinical points follows for the major groups of medication.

◆ *Antipsychotics*
• usually safe to give, but the traditional agents have effects on most neurotransmitter systems, so side-effects abound
• many medical/surgical staff have not seen, or will be slower to recognize **neuroleptic malignant syndrome**, **dystonic reactions**, **akathisia** and **pseudoparkinsonism**
• newer antipsychotics are not available in parenteral forms

◆ *Anticholinergic Agents*
• staff may need instruction on what to look for and how to give these medications (i.e., IM injection in severe cases)
• anticholinergic effects are additive to the effects of the antipsychotics, which can lead to **anticholingeric toxicity**
• akathisia does not respond to this group of medications

◆ *Antidepressants*
• while frequently prescribed, the delay in onset of action requires use after discharge, so you need to involve the G.P.
• older agents have more side effects and induce more manic episodes in patients with Bipolar Mood Disorder; these drugs have many clinical uses that newer agents (currently) don't
• newer antidepressants are better tolerated and much safer when taken in overdose, but are more expensive and may be stigmatized because of the popularity of Prozac®

◆ *Mood Stabilizers*
• all require blood levels and organ system monitoring
• may affect the efficacy of other medications (e.g. hepatic metabolism induction by carbamazepine)
• there is a delayed onset of action for mood symptom control
• anticonvulsants have a significant risk of teratogenesis
• lithium needs to be given cautiously to patients who are not adequately hydrated (e.g. post-op, NPO); levels should be drawn 12h after the last dose

◆ Antianxiety Agents
- benzodiazepines are the most commonly prescribed drugs in this category, but others can be used (e.g. buspirone, propranolol, some tricyclic antidepressants, hydroxyzine, etc.)
- the longer the half-life of the medication, the more it will affect daytime alertness (i.e. "a hangover" effect); on the other hand, shorter acting compounds have a higher abuse potential due to rebound anxiety
- lorazepam, oxazepam and temazepam are rapidly metabolized by direct conjugation and do not have active metabolites — these are important considerations in patients with liver disease (e.g. due to alcohol dependence)

◆ Hypnotics
- again, benzodiazepines are popular but can lead to dependence if given for a period longer than two weeks
- REM cycles are affected by benzodiazepines
- other medications are available (e.g. chloral hydrate, zolpidem, zopiclone)
- discussing sleep hygiene with patients may reduce or remove the need for medications; many people sleep poorly in hospital due to the noise, strange bed, roommates, etc.

◆ Stimulants
- may need to be given to those who have treatment-resistant depression
- patients who are receiving palliative care and have become depressed may be candidates due to the speed of onset and efficacy of these medications in elevating mood

◆ General Considerations
- because many referring physicians treat illnesses with medications, they often expect you to prescribe *something*
- because patients receive a number of medications in hospital, be vigilant for potential interactions
- you are the primary source of information for psychotropic medications (and for obtaining consent), a few moments spent explaining such matters can be very helpful

The Consult Report & Recommendations

D/ Longer-Term Medication Considerations

Outlining longer-term medication considerations is usually not done in the initial consult note. These factors become relevant as the admission progresses and when the patient's response to your original recommendations is known.

If you are going to see the person once or only for a short time, it is helpful to include a management outline. For example, if a patient is being started on lithium, you might include the following helpful points in your note:

- reminders about measuring drug levels and when to do so (e.g. 4 — 7 days after a dosage change)
- the serum range for acute treatment
- lab indices to monitor (e.g. a leukocytosis may occur)

Other general considerations include:

- if the medication should be continued upon discharge
- if you will be following the patient or will contact the G.P. to offer advice on the long term use
- if alternate preparations are available or should be considered (e.g. suspensions instead of pills, depot forms of neuroleptics, sustained-release tablets) and possible dosing arrangements (e.g. once daily, bid, tid, etc.)

References for Psychotropic Drug Information

These resources are particularly useful in C-L psychiatry:

Psychotropic Drugs Fast Facts, Second Edition
J.S. Maxmen & N.G. Ward
W. W. Norton & Co., New York, 1995

Biological Therapies in Psychiatry Newsletter
A.J. Gelenberg, Editor
Gelenberg Consulting & Publishing, Tucson, AZ

Clinical Handbook of Psychotropic Drugs, Ninth Edition
K.Z. Bezchlibnyk-Butler, J.J. Jeffries & B.A. Martin, Editors
Hogrefe & Huber Publishers, Seattle, 1999

E/ Psychological/Psychotherapeutic Treatments

While referring teams may modify your suggested biological investigations and treatments, there is usually little objection to your recommending and implementing a form of psychotherapy with patients. As long as your sessions don't unduly upset patients or interfere with other treatments, consultees are almost always grateful that you will share your time and expertise.

The range of treatments available overall is impressive and expanding. Most of the letters in the **"ABCDEFGHIJKLMN"** mnemonic (page 121) are forms of psychotherapy. However, not all of these modalities will be available or advisable for inpatients.

The approaches most applicable to C-L psychiatry are usually:

- brief
- reality-based
- solution-focused
- cognitive or educational in nature

It is usually sufficient to record in the recommendation section that ongoing psychotherapy is indicated and that either you will be doing it or will speak with the person who will. You can mention the type of therapy involved and briefly state the goals that are appropriate for this intervention. This is especially important if the patient is engaging in behavior that is problematic for the primary physician. Here, "consultation" psychiatry provides psychotherapy for the patient while "liaison" psychiatry also helps the referring team. Personality-disordered patients can, through the use of unconscious ego defense mechanisms, elicit strong responses from referring teams. For example, **projection** may engender hostile responses towards patients, while **splitting** may cause some consultees to behave seductively.

F/ Social Treatments

Social treatments focus on assisting patients with working and living arrangements. For example, patients who have had accidents or who have chronic psychiatric illnesses may need vocational rehabilitation during or after hospital stays. Some patients will require help in finding shelters or group homes. While there are usually social workers or other staff to assist with these matters, keeping abreast of community agencies and supports is important. Often there are directories available listing various resources. Social treatments can also involve linking patients with local or national self-help groups. A listing of useful articles is provided in McCartney (1985).

Documenting the Consultation

The consultation note has to include a number of essential pieces of information for academic, financial, research and clinical reasons, yet be brief enough to be useful to consultees. Recently, two articles have been written which provide further guidance regarding consult notes. The sample C-L note provided in this chapter contains the recommendations set out by Bronheim (1998) in the APM Practice Guidelines, though three points bear emphasis: avoid using acronyms and jargon, remember that records are available to third parties, and consult notes must be signed.

Worley et al (1998) provide a structured C-L Form that complies with **Health Care Financing Administration (HCFA)** and **American Medical Association (AMA)** Guidelines. The authors warn that severe financial penalties can be levied if physicians' documentation cannot justify the services that have been billed.

Sample Consultation Notes

The next section contains three medical notes:

- a medical admission note outlining the physical aspects of a patient's illness; this is often the only source of information on the hospital record at the time of the consult
- an "overly psychiatric" consultation note which provides a considerable amount of detail, but doesn't address key issues that referring teams would find helpful
- a balanced psychiatric consultation note which blends data from both of the above sources into a coherent summary and which outlines a treatment plan based on the guidelines listed in this chapter

Sigmundoscopy — The Bases

MEDICAL ADMISSION NOTE

by Dr. Billy Rubin
Dept. of Medicine PGY-2
May 5th

Information obtained from patient interview & old chart.

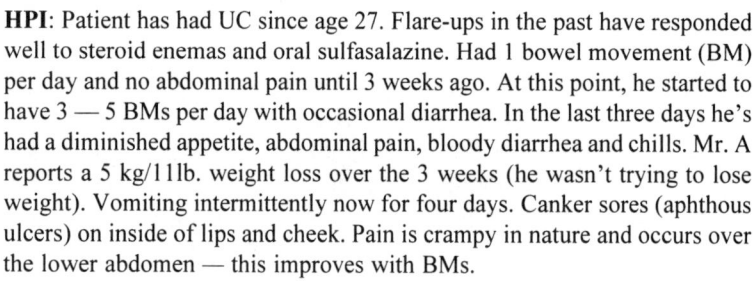

ID: Mr A is a 32y male old teacher.

RFA: Exacerbation of ulcerative colitis (UC).

HPI: Patient has had UC since age 27. Flare-ups in the past have responded well to steroid enemas and oral sulfasalazine. Had 1 bowel movement (BM) per day and no abdominal pain until 3 weeks ago. At this point, he started to have 3 — 5 BMs per day with occasional diarrhea. In the last three days he's had a diminished appetite, abdominal pain, bloody diarrhea and chills. Mr. A reports a 5 kg/11lb. weight loss over the 3 weeks (he wasn't trying to lose weight). Vomiting intermittently now for four days. Canker sores (aphthous ulcers) on inside of lips and cheek. Pain is crampy in nature and occurs over the lower abdomen — this improves with BMs.

Denies having any arthralgias, eye problems, liver involvement or skin problems. No recent travel or unusual foods. Very stressed at work lately.

HPH: UC (5 years ago)
Gastroesophageal reflux (10 years)
Benign familial tremor
Sigmoid polypectomy (1 year ago — benign)

Meds: sulfasalazine 2 g p.o. daily
loperamide 2 mg caps p.o. prn
codeine phosphate 30 mg p.o. qid

Allergies: Environmental (ragweed and pollen); none to drugs

Personal: Home-room teacher for grade 6. Never married, lives with parents. Bachelor's degree in Arts, then attended Teacher's College. His alcohol intake is minimal and he doesn't imbibe during flare-ups. Last drink was 4 weeks ago. Non-smoker, doesn't use recreational drugs.

Family: Parents and 1 younger sister all alive — none have UC. Family history of heart disease, but no known incidence of cancer (esp. bowel). Parents have had screening colonoscopies which have been normal.

The Consult Report & Recommendations

Physical Exam:
Alert, oriented and stable. Looks pale. Seems anxious and upset at times.

Vitals: BP 130/80, HR 80 and regular, RR 14, T = 38 C

HEENT: pupils equal and reactive to light; no papilledema; full extra-ocular movements; ears clear; several aphthous ulcers; mucous membranes dry

Chest: clear to IPPA, no wheezes or crackles, good air entry

CVS: $S_1 S_2$ — regular rhythm, systolic ejection murmur, no elevation in JVP, peripheral pulses palpable

Abdomen: no scars or asymmetry; LKKS not palpable; no masses, bowel sounds present; DRE deferred until settled   *tenderness to deep palpation*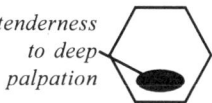

Neuro/MSK: CN 2 — 12 intact; no sensory deficits, DTRs are normal; no Babinski; gait is normal; cerebellar testing is WNL

Labs: $\dfrac{135 \ | \ 3.5}{98 \ | \ 30} < \dfrac{3.6}{60}$ *Blood Counts:* $10.5 \ 118 \curlyvee 396$

ESR 80, INR 1.2, PTT 26
LFTs, RFTs, calcium, magnesium, phosphate, albumin pending
Stool C & S, blood C & S to be taken on arrival to floor

Impression: 32 year old man with history of UC for 7 years. Has had episodic flare-ups over this time. Well until 3 weeks ago when he developed increased frequency of BMs with occasional diarrhea. Now acutely ill for 3 — 4 days with abdo pain, blood in diarrhea and chills — all consistent with another flare-up. Oral intake is poor due to aphthous ulcers and vomiting, which has led to an 11 lb. weight loss and dehydration at present. No involvement of joints, eyes, skin or liver/biliary tract at present. Compliance with medication is good.

Pt. anxious and upset during interview and examination — feels stressed at work.

Plan:
- Admit to medical team
- Rehydrate and give IV corticosteroids
- Monitor hemoglobin daily
- Arrange flexible sigmoidoscopy/colonoscopy
- Consult General Surgery and Psychiatry

PSYCHIATRIC CONSULTATION NOTE

by Dr. S. Froyd
Dept. of Psychoanalysis
May 6th 9:00 a.m.

Information obtained from:
Patient Interview

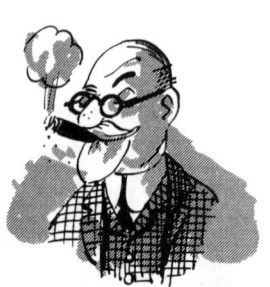

Mr. A is a 32 year-old, single, male, public school teacher who was referred for psychiatric consultation during an admission for exacerbation of ulcerative colitis. Mr. A's internist explained that he complained of depressive and anxious symptoms which he felt were related to stress at work. Mr. A's job has become more demanding as his class size increased and students with disturbed behavior and borderline normal intelligence have been included in the regular classes. Mr. A struggles to control the class' behavior and to maintain reasonable academic standards under these difficult conditions. This is a special challenge for Mr. A who tends to have high standards for himself and who is not comfortable with situations which he feels he can't control. The recent exacerbation of ulcerative colitis appears to be associated with Mr. A's feeling that he did not have his principal's support in attempting to deal with the misbehavior of two boys in the class. Mr. A appears highly motivated to get the principal's approval by controlling the class' behavior and successfully completing the academic program. This has been difficult because of the disruptive behavior of these students, whom the principal will not suspend for more than three days. Mr. A appears to struggle between his wish to please the principal and his increasing resentment at the principal for not helping him deal with the situation. His anxiety increases whenever he becomes aware of his anger at the principal.

Mr. A's parents were blue collar workers who had high expectations of him. He has a younger sister who was expected to complete high school, get married and raise a family, which she did. Mr. A's father, a retired factory worker, wanted him to succeed in a profession which his father felt would bring prestige to the family and justify the sacrifices in putting Mr. A through university. Mr. A described his father as strict, de-

The Consult Report & Recommendations

Psychiatric Consultation
Dr. S. Froyd
Page 2

manding and quite involved. Mr. A's father used to be pleased when Mr. A got high marks, but would express dissatisfaction at anything less than honors, and expected Mr. A to have a part-time job during high school to help pay for his university education. Mr. A felt all of this to be a considerable demand, although he was anxious to please his father. He described his mother in generally positive terms, as being less demanding than his father and reasonably affectionate. However, she worked at night and was to some extent unavailable to Mr. A except on weekends and holidays.

Mr. A dated a number of women since leaving university, but hasn't had a relationship last for more than 12 months. He feels that women find him rather fussy and inflexible. A couple of them have indicated that they felt that he was not ready to leave his parents and make a commitment to marriage. The closest relationship he's had was with a woman whom he dated for 10 months at the age of 27. In spite of some ambivalence on his part, he was prepared to marry her when she unexpectedly broke off their relationship, complaining that he was still too attached to his parents. This separation was followed by the onset of bloody diarrhea and abdominal pain, with an eventual diagnosis of ulcerative colitis.

Mr. A has always lived with his parents, except for one year when he attended university in another city. This was a difficult year for him as he did not make many friends while away. He kept in almost constant telephone contact with his parents and frequently flew back for weekend visits and all holidays. Mr. A appears to have internalized his father's demanding attitude towards him, with the result that he has quite a demanding attitude towards himself. He appears to project his internal image of his father onto his principal, wishing to please the principal under circumstances which seem to be as demanding as those that he grew up with. He appears to deal with his resentment towards the principal with a reaction formation, and instead tries to please the principal. This resentment likely

Psychiatric Consultation
Dr. S. Froyd
Page 3

is amplified by his repressed resentment towards his father, whom the principal appears to represent for Mr. A.

Mr. A appears to have had some difficulty in separating from his parents and establishing close adult relationships. In particular, he has had difficulty in developing his own standards and ideals, and instead appears to have persisted in attempting to fulfill his father's standards in order to get his father's approval. This may be understood on the basis of his father's withholding approval unless Mr. A functioned at a very high level, on the many demands Mr. A's father made of him, and on his mother's relative unavailability. The onset and exacerbation of episodes of colitis appears related to frustrations and losses in relationships which Mr. A has not felt able to control. These include the breakup of his relationship with his girlfriend and the present difficulty with his principal, with whom he is frustrated and cannot express his anger, but whom he wants to please. This likely is a repetition of the pattern he experienced over the years with his father. Mr. A's mother's unavailability likely has made him more vulnerable to separation.

Diagnostic Impression: Adjustment Disorder with Mixed Emotional Features; Psychological Factors Affecting Physical Disorders; Personality Disorder with Obsessive-Compulsive and Dependent traits.

Plan: Mr. A's symptoms do not appear to warrant the prescription of a psychoactive medication. This consultant will interview him on a regular basis while he is in hospital in an attempt to establish a psychotherapeutic relationship. If Mr. A is amenable, the consultant will arrange to meet with him on a thrice-weekly basis for 50 minutes in order to begin a supportive psychotherapy in which Mr. A can explore the difficulties he is having with his principal and how these difficulties may be related to the exacerbation of his colitis. Depending on the outcome of this therapy, a more ambitious psychodynamic therapy may be attempted.

The Consult Report & Recommendations

Psychiatric Consultation Note
by Dr. B. Eager, Pager 0968/Ext. 2094
PGY-3, C-L Psychiatry Service
May 6th   2:30 p.m. — 4:00 p.m.

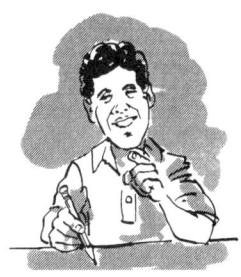

Information obtained from: patient interview and hospital chart
Consult requested by: Dr. G. I. Joe

I.D. Mr. A is a 32 year old, white, single, male public school teacher currently living with his parents.

Reason for Admission Mr. A was admitted May 5th due to a flare-up of ulcerative colitis (UC) during which he became increasingly ill over a 3 week period. He was diagnosed with UC 7 years ago and has required 4 inpatient stays in this time period.

Reason for Referral Evaluation of depressive and anxious symptoms; provide continuing care while in hospital; advise on suitability of outpatient follow-up. Referral received May 6th.

History of Present Illness Mr. A was last well about 3 weeks ago. At that time, he started to experience a change in bowel habits which intensified into a systemic resurgence of his illness. He was dehydrated on admission and has a sigmoidoscopy booked for later today.

His illness has taken a toll on him emotionally, and he was noted to be "anxious and upset" during the admission interview and physical. Mr. A is currently the homeroom teacher for a Grade 6 class. He devotes a considerable amount of his time preparing lessons that "meet the letter" of the education objectives. Since the holidays, his class size has increased because several families relocated near his school. A special education teacher left and students with borderline normal intelligence were also added to his class. The increased number of students, and in particular those requiring extra attention, have disrupted his usual careful planning. Mr. A likes to have the full attention of the class, and is aware that control issues are important to him. About the time of the onset of his symptoms, two boys released a handful of insects in the class, which disrupted the entire afternoon and required a pest control company to be involved. The students were suspended by the principal for three days, which is far less than the two weeks Mr. A had requested. Mr. A has worked diligently to impress the principal, and has distinguished himself. This has been the only disagreement so far.

Psychiatric Consultation — Page 2
Dr. B. Eager/C-L Psychiatry Service

Evaluation of depressive symptoms is as follows:
- **sleep** — has had trouble with initial insomnia for 3 weeks, no early morning awakening, no sedative medications
- **appetite** — diminished with flare-up, has lost 11 lbs. in 3 weeks (not desired); usually a picky eater (avoids dairy products)
- **mood** — describes it as down persistently for 3 days; gives himself a score of 3/10 and is usually a 7 or 8
- **interest** — able to stay up with demands of school; reads newspapers and novels; less enthusiastic this week only
- **concentration** — unimpaired; able to recall 3/3 objects, serial 7's all correct, spelled "WORLD" backwards properly
- **guilt/worthlessness** — describes these as continual issues for him, but no worse at this time
- **psychomotor changes** — not observable during the interview
- **energy** — plays squash twice-weekly; hasn't played this week due to physical condition, but otherwise energy level described as normal
- **suicide** — no thoughts of harm to self or others; no past attempts

Evaluation of anxious symptoms is as follows:
- anxiety is episodic, and almost always clearly related to identifiable factors; in this situation, he is concerned about his performance as a teacher and the outcome of this flare-up (e.g. will he need surgery?)
- his feelings of anxiousness last for up to 6 weeks, but vary according to the cycles of exams and teacher evaluations
- doesn't describe discrete obsessions or compulsions, but has a pervasive drive to achieve high standards in all facets of his life
- no discrete panic attacks or life-threatening experiences
- not afraid to go places where help/escape not easily arranged
- not solely concerned with humiliation or embarrassment
- his fear is not cued by certain objects or situations

Review of Symptoms No complaints or observations consistent with psychotic disorders, bipolar mood disorder, hypochondriasis, eating disorders or substance abuse/dependence.

Psychiatric History No psychiatric admissions. He saw a counselor on two occasions in university (for exam stress) and was given sleeping medication which was effective; Mr. A drinks socially, doesn't smoke cigarettes and denies current or past substance abuse.

Medications sulfasalazine 2 g p.o. daily; loperamide 2 mg caps p.o. prn; codeine phosphate 30 mg p.o. qid; over-the-counter sleeping pills

Psychiatric Consultation — Page 3
Dr. B. Eager/C-L Psychiatry Service

Medical History Other than having UC, Mr. A is healthy. In high school, he was knocked unconscious for under 10 seconds in a football game.

Personal/Social History Mr. A was told he had an unremarkable birth. He met his developmental milestones appropriately. He attended school at age 5, which was age appropriate. He did well in school and did not need remedial help at any point. He idealized one of his primary school teachers (a former athlete) and gives this as a partial reason for his occupation. Mr. A is exclusively heterosexual and began to date in late high school. Long-term relationships have been difficult for him — he describes his girlfriends as pushing him too much to leave his parents' house and make a commitment. He has never been married. Mr. A left home for one year of university and then sought employment only in his hometown. He describes himself as always trying to make his parents proud and felt they would be more interested and kept up to date on his progress if he lived in the same city.

Other than one speeding ticket, Mr. A has no current legal difficulties, and has never been charged with an offense. He has not been involved in military service.

Family History Mr. A is not aware of any members of his immediate family having been diagnosed with a psychiatric disorder. He recalls certain stress-related problems his father had, especially at times of union contract negotiations and promotions. His extended family was similarly reported to be free of psychiatric difficulties as far as he knew.

Mental Status Exam
- Appearance — well groomed, wearing hospital pajamas
- Behavior — fidgeted and looked out the window at times, otherwise calm
- Speech/Thought Form — no abnormalities detected (NAD)
- Thought Content — centered on school concerns and fear of surgery
- Affect & Mood — as described above
- Perception — NAD
- Insight & Judgment — deemed intact on the basis of his awareness of his illness and appropriate actions to get help; he is willing to go along with the recommendations of his attending physician and listed the major long-term complications of UC and the risks of not receiving treatment
- Cognitive Functions — oriented x 3; registration, recent and remote recall intact; general knowledge intact; concentration and attention as described

Psychiatric Consultation — Page 4
Dr. B. Eager/C-L Psychiatry Service

Summary Mr. A is a 32 year old man admitted for a flare-up of UC, his 4th admission in 7 years. He relates the onset of a variety of mood and anxiety symptoms to the situation at work and the worsening of his physical state. He has a history of difficulty coping with situations that seem beyond his control and that may reflect negatively on him (especially tests and evaluations). Using DSM-IV criteria, he does not appear to have a major mood or anxiety disorder at this time.

Diagnostic Impression
Axis I: Adjustment Disorder With Mixed Anxiety and Depressed Mood
Axis II: Obsessive-Compulsive & Dependent Personality Traits
Axis III: Ulcerative Colitis
Differential Diagnosis: Depression, Generalized Anxiety Disorder

Treatment Recommendations for the Referring Team
• Suggest a TSH level & a folate level be drawn (due to sulfasalazine)
• A benzodiazepine (lorazepam 1mg or oxazepam 15mg) p.o. qhs can replace his sleeping medication (unknown at present)
• Given that he doesn't currently appear to have a clear-cut mood or anxiety disorder, a psychotropic medication is not indicated; agents useful in both these conditions (i.e. SSRIs & TCAs) can cause GI upset which may aggravate his condition and make it difficult to sort out whether it was his UC or the medication making him ill
• Because of the clear association between work-related stress and the seriousness of his flare-up, a complete resolution is advisable before he returns to work — suggest a medical leave of absence

Recommended Treatment by the C-L Team
• Mr. A is a suitable candidate for short-term psychotherapy which can begin this week if he is agreeable
• Our team will contact the school (with Mr. A's permission) to see if his performance has justifiably caused concern there

Reference
E.A. Walker, M.D. Gelfand, A.N. Gelfand, F. Creed & W. J. Katon
The Relationship of Current Psychiatric Disorder to Functional Disability and Distress in Patients with Inflammatory Bowel Disease
General Hospital Psychiatry 18(4): p. 220 — 229, 1996

The Consult Report & Recommendations

Critique of the Three Notes
◆ The medical note is a "bare bones" record of the admission outlining almost exclusively the physical aspects of the illness. There is a brief notation in the HPI and another in the physical exam section pertaining to the patient's emotional status. This is not an uncommon amount of documentation for a referral made early in the admission — the medical resident knew there was a need for a psychiatric consult.

◆ The note by Dr. Froyd is a good, thorough, psychodynamically relevant document. Unfortunately, it misses the mark as a good consult note because several key areas are not addressed, even though the consult question is answered. This is a common pitfall among psychiatric residents (and consultants) who think that the referring source is as interested in psychiatry as they are, and that every factoid of information should be included.

◆ The note by Dr. Eager is a complete and satisfactory consult report. It embodies all of the elements discussed in this chapter though it is necessarily less detailed in certain areas than Dr. Froyd's note. Breaking down the various sections helps a busy physician identify which sections he or she would like to read. There is a thorough cataloging of diagnostic criteria for the two conditions listed in the reason for referral. This not only illustrates the rationale for the diagnostic impression, it allows you to follow the progress of specific symptoms during your visits. Although there were few findings on the MSE, it was still performed and documented. Two features of medical relevance were discovered during the interview: the use of an over-the-counter sleeping medication and a distant head injury. The recommendations include consideration of biopsychosocial factors both for investigations and treatment. The suggested folate level was made after reading the particulars about this medication. The reference is from a psychiatry journal, not a medical one, which could be seen as implying that the referring source doesn't stay current with the literature. In some cases, the goals for psychotherapy may be omitted or given in more detail depending on confidentiality considerations and the interest of the referring source.

Summary

Psychiatric consultation reports answer two main questions:

- What is going on with the patient?
- What can be done about it?

A consult request in a sense forms a "contract" with explicit and implicit obligations. The consult note documents your opinion/answers to the above questions and outlines management suggestions. A suggested outline for reports is as follows:

- A clearly-written title, and in a prominent section includes your name, position, pager/phone extension and the referring source
- Time, date, length of interview; sources of information
- Identifying features of the patient
- A synopsis of the patient's medical illness and course
- Reason for the referral/Expectations of the consultee
- Outline of the biopsychosocial factors leading up to the consult
- Detailed inquiry into factors related to the consult question
- Review of symptoms for other psychiatric illnesses
- Psychiatric history (including psychotherapy & medications)
- Medications, allergies, substance use
- Personal, social & family history; legal history; military history
- Mental status examination
- Summary/Impression/Formulation with diagnosis and differential
- Recommendations/Suggestions
- References or articles

If the above list constitutes the "science" of writing a note, the "art" balances the following factors:

thorough documentation	vs.	interest level of the consultee
emphasis on detail	vs.	emphasis on confidentiality
technical jargon	vs.	precision in phenomenology
explaining rationale for recommendations	vs.	"just do it" implementation
thorough investigations for physical causes	vs.	the expense and relatively low yield of abnormal results

References

S.A. Cohen-Cole, in
Consultation Psychitary: A Practical Guide
R. Michels, J.O. Cavenar & A.M. Cooper, Editors
Lippincott, Philadelphia, 1988

T.N. Garrick & N.L. Stotland
How To Write A Psychiatric Consultation
American Journal of Psychiatry 139(7): p. 849 — 855, 1982

R.C.W. Hall, E.R. Gardner, S.K. Stickney, A.F. LeCann et al
Physical Illness Manifesting as Psychiatric Illness
Archives of General Psychiatry 37: p. 989 — 995, 1980

C.F. McCartney, D.L. Evans & W. Richardson
Library Collection of the Psychosocial Publications in Consultation-Liaison Psychiatry
General Hospital Psychiatry 7(1): p. 73 — 82, 1985

M.L. Popkin, T.B. Mackenzie, R.C.W. Hall & A.L. Callies
Consultees' Concordance With Consultant's Psychotropic Drug Recommendations
Archives of General Psychiatry 37: p. 1017 — 1021, 1980

M.L. Popkin, T.B. Mackenzie, A.L. Callies et al
Yield of Psychiatric Consultants' Recommendations for Diagnostic Action
Archives of General Psychiatry 39: p. 843 — 845, 1982

M.L. Popkin, T.B. Mackenzie & A.L. Callies
Consultation-Liaison Outcome Evaluation
Archives of General Psychiatry 40: p. 215 — 219, 1983

N. L. Stotland & T.R. Garrick
Manual of Psychiatric Consultation
American Psychiatric Press, Inc. Washington, D.C., 1990

Z. Taintor, J. Spikes, L.H. Gise & J.J. Strain
Recording Psychiatric Consultations: A Preliminary Report
General Hospital Psychiatry 1(2): p. 139 — 149, 1979

Sigmundoscopy — The Bases

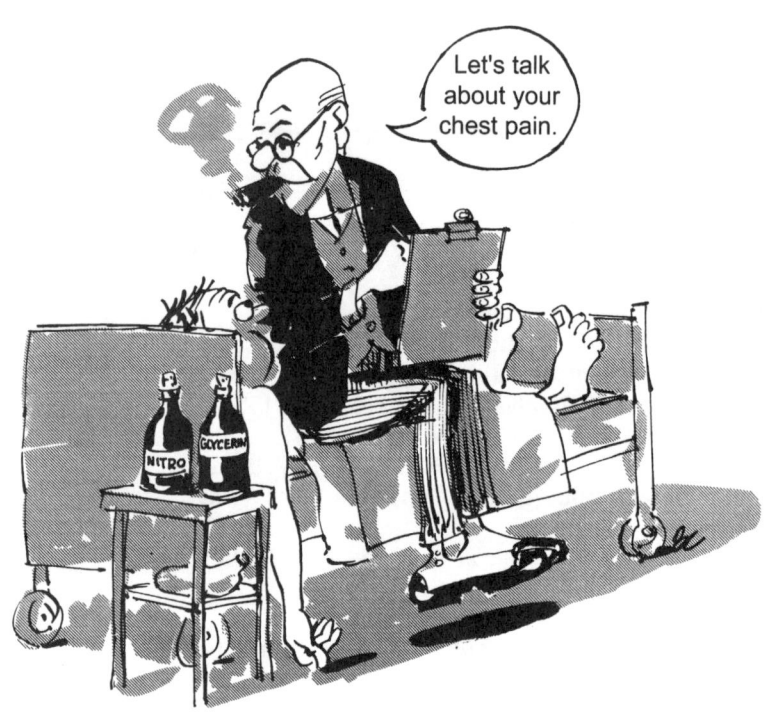

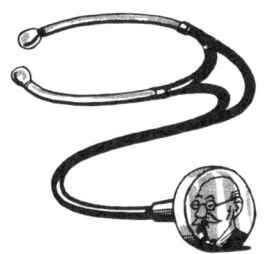

5/ Implementing the Treatment Plan

The two previous chapters have outlined the first four stages in the process of conducting a psychiatric consultation.

- **The Referral**
- **Preparing for the Consult**
- **Interviewing the Patient**
- **Writing the Consult Report**
- **Implementing the Treatment Plan**

A thorough interview and a well-written note are key factors in providing psychiatric consultation. However, an appropriate or even elegant treatment plan doesn't benefit the patient until your recommendations are implemented by the referring source. The degree to which consultees implement the recommendations in your treatment plan has been termed **concordance**, a discussion of which is presented in this chapter. The subject of concordance is discussed in detail, focusing on such areas as:

- what level of concordance is expectable?
- does the level of concordance vary with the type of recommendation made?
- does the status of the person doing the consult matter?
- why would consultees not implement recommendations?
- do other specialist consultants have similar problems?
- what can be done to increase the degree of concordance?

Concordance

At this point in the consult process, you have taken care of the preliminary process matters outlined in the previous two chapters, interviewed the patient and informed the referring source of your recommendations via your consult note, and potentially with an after-consult discussion. You return the next day to check on the patient's progress and find that none of your suggestions were implemented. You are not even sure if the primary physician read your note as there is no "thank you" followed by a set of initials, as is a popular practice. Your visit with the patient also reveals that the treating team made no mention of your plan at rounds.

Does this happen often? Is it you? Something you suggested? Or are they just getting around to your note and will give it due consideration when they have the chance? Should you contact the team to ask why, speak to a supervisor or colleague, or just wait it out? These and other salient matters will be dealt with in this section, which reviews some of the literature on this topic.

Popkin, Mackenzie et al published a series of articles between 1979 and 1983 in a number of journals that explored various aspects of the implementation of psychiatric consultant's recommendations. They developed terminology that was used by other authors in subsequent articles:

• **concordance** was used to describe the degree of implementation of consult recommendations; the authors felt this term described the mutuality of the consultation interchange rather than the unilateral connotation of the term "compliance" (in this chapter concordance, compliance and implementation are used interchangeably)

• **representation** is the presence of the psychiatric diagnosis/diagnoses on the medical discharge summary

The following sections summarize reports on various aspects of concordance with accompanying references. Because there are discrepancies between studies, for the sake of clarity and brevity, the emphasis here is on the positive findings (i.e. where something significant was found) from these reports.

CLOES

CLOES is an acronym for **Consultation-Liaison Outcome Evaluation System**, which was developed by Popkin, Mackenzie et al. Their series of articles provides a set of standardized criteria to measure concordance. CLOES criteria are listed here in an abbreviated form to provide a frame of reference to be able to interpret the results. Criteria for **concordance (C)**, **partial concordance (PC)** and **nonconcordance (NC)** were developed to measure three major areas of study:

- **Compliance with psychotropic medication suggestions**
    - C — if started within 96 hours and the dosage was between 75 and 125% of that recommended
    - PC — if started within 96 hours and a dosage of between 50 to 74% or 126 to 150% of that recommended was used
    - NC — advised drug or equivalent not used within 96 hours in the absence of contraindications for doing so

- **Representation of consultants' psychiatric diagnoses**
    - C — if a verbatim or near-verbatim representation was made
    - PC — an uncertain representation was made
    - NC — no mention of the diagnosis was made

- **Implementation of recommendations for diagnostic action**
    - C — if the recommended action was implemented within 96 hours; if multiple recommendations were made, over 75% of them were carried out
    - PC — if multiple recommendations were made and between 50 to 74% of them were followed
    - NC — if the recommended action was not carried out, or in the case of multiple recommendations, less than 50% were carried out

In many studies, the PC category was re-scored or dropped from the analysis to gain a clearer appreciation for which variables were associated with C or NC outcomes. The criteria are fully listed in:

M.L. Popkin, T.B. Mackenzie & A.L. Callies
Consultation-Liaison Outcome Evaluation
Archives of General Psychiatry 40: p. 215 — 219, 1983

◆ Concordance for Medication Recommendations

Popkin, Mackenzie et al began with a retrospective look at the degree of implementation for psychiatric consultant's medication suggestions. Their results were as follows:

- 200 consults were reviewed, with psychotropic medication recommendations being made in (55%) of cases
- Implementation was 68% C, 11% PC and 24% NC

They found that there were significant differences among the different actions involving medications, which were:

- stop   93%
- adjust   90%
- continue (as taken prior to admission) 80%
- start   68%

When a dosage was specified, concordance in starting medication was 68% vs. 46% when it was not. Overall, consultees started medications at about 80% of the recommended dosage.

A second study was conducted to further determine related variables. They found statistically higher concordance levels where:

- a medication was either adjusted, continued or stopped (these actions formed a separate "non-start" group as the action of "starting" a medication has a lower concordance)
- multiple recommendations were made
- the consult occurred in the first half of the admission
- the patient had a history of taking, or was currently using, a psychotropic medication
- the recommendation to start a medication was accompanied by a specified dosage (this was particularly so if the consultation note was shorter)

A study by Neill (1979) found that there were differences between types of recommended medications, with antipsychotics being concordant 90% of the time vs. 65% for benzodiazepines and 56% for tricyclic antidepressants. Huyse et al (1993) found that 77% of consults included a medication suggestion, and he concurred with the finding that medication recommendations made earlier in the hospital stay had a greater chance of implementation. Billowitz (1979) found that the referring service had differing compliance rates (with Medicine > Ob/Gyn > Surgery).

Summary
Referring physicians may exhibit a dichotomy in prescribing psychotropic medications in that they see a patient as someone who either would or would not use them. Previous or current use of psychotropics seems to make it easier for consultees to implement recommendations for drug treatments. The reason for referral may affect concordance in that psychotic or disruptive patients are more likely to be given medication. Familiarity with psychotropic medication or a higher degree of overlap between psychiatry and the referring specialty (e.g. Medicine > Surgery) increases concordance for medication suggestions. The changing agendas during a patient's stay influence the timing of consult requests, as well as the receptiveness to medication suggestions.

References for Medication Concordance
A. Billowitz & W. Friedson
Are Psychiatric Consultants' Recommendations Followed?
Internat. J. of Psychiatry in Medicine 9(2): p. 179 — 189, 1978-79

F.J. Huyse, J.S. Lyons & J.J. Strain
The Sequencing of Psychiatric Recommendations
Psychosomatics 34: p. 307 — 313, 1993

J.R. Neill
Consultation Evaluation: I. Psychotropic Drug Recommendations
General Hospital Psychiatry April 1(1): p. 62 — 65, 1979

M.L. Popkin, T.B. Mackenzie, R.C.W. Hall & J.G. Garrard
Physicians' Concordance With Consultant's Recommendations For Psychotropic Medication
Archives of General Psychiatry 36: p. 386 — 389, 1979

M.L. Popkin, T.B. Mackenzie, R.C.W. Hall & A.L. Callies
Consultees' Concordance With Consultants' Psychotropic Drug Recommendations
Archives of General Psychiatry 37: p. 1017 — 1021, 1979

◆ Concordance for Diagnostic Actions

Popkin (1980) reported that:

- in 29% of their consults they suggested diagnostic action(s)
- the overall concordance for their cases was 53%

Then, he grouped the diagnostic actions into four subtypes and reported the concordance based on individual recommendations:

- consultations (from other services)   67%
- diagnostic procedures/exams   65%
- laboratory determinations   61%
- psychological testing   54%

The two most frequent recommendations in each category were (respectively):

- neurology & endocrinology   (consultations)
- EEGs & EKGs   (diag. procedures)
- thyroid & other clinical chemistry tests   (lab. tests)
- personality & cognitive testing   (psych. testing)

The difference in rates of concordance between these four groups was not statistically significant. Concordance was found to be higher in the following circumstances:

- as the age of the patient increased (especially > 60 years)
- with the diagnosis of an **organic mental disorder (OMD)**
- the longer the period of hospitalization after the consult
- with longer-term admissions

In a second study, Popkin (1982) looked at the prevalence of abnormal results for psychiatrists' diagnostic recommendations and found an overall yield of 45%. Patients with OMDs had the greatest likelihood of having an abnormal result (81%). The tests with the highest yield of abnormal results were:

- MMPI   76%
- EEG   69%
- thyroid function tests   52%
- vitamin B_{12} level   47%
- folate level   44%

Huyse (1993) reported concordance rates of 58% and 55% for biological diagnostic actions and psychosocial actions respectively, which agrees with Popkin's results. Huyse's results indicated that psychosocial diagnostic actions were more likely to be implemented during an admission. In another study, Huyse (1990) found that diagnostic recommendations for actions that varied from the consultees' usual activities were less likely to be carried out. In particular, obtaining psychosocial information from general practitioners and families were the investigations with the lowest yields (40% and 52%). Popkin (1980) found that a follow-up note on the chart increased concordance.

Summary

A consistent finding in these studies was a concordance rate of less than 60% for investigations, despite the relatively high yield of abnormal results when recommendations were implemented. Popkin (1982) suggested that once referring sources determine that a patient's problem is psychiatric, the evaluative process terminates. Higher concordance rates later in an admission may be related to the complexity of the case and/or the perplexity of the consultee. Overall, referring sources are more interested in management recommendations than in evaluative ones.

References for Diagnostic Action Recommendations

F.J. Huyse, J.J. Strain & J.S. Hammer
Interventions in C-L Psychiatry, Part II: Concordance
General Hospital Psychiatry 12: p. 221 — 231, 1990

F.J. Huyse, J.S. Lyons & J.J. Strain
The Sequencing of Psychiatric Recommendations
Psychosomatics 34: p. 307 — 313, 1993

M.L. Popkin, T.B. Mackenzie, & A.L. Callies
Consultees' Concordance With Consultants' Recommendations For Diagnostic Action
Journal of Nervous and Mental Disorders 168(1): p. 9 — 12, 1980

M.L. Popkin, T.B. Mackenzie, A.L. Callies & R.C.W. Hall
Yield of Psychiatric Consultants' Recommendations for Diagnostic Action
Archives of General Psychiatry 39: p. 843 — 845, 1982

◆ Diagnostic Representation

Callies (1980) looked at the incorporation of psychiatric diagnoses (**representation**) in the medical/surgical discharge summary from the initial consult note. After dropping PC cases from the evaluation, the overall concordance rate was 50%. Factors significantly related to concordance were:

> • the primary medical diagnosis at discharge; if the patient's difficulties were deemed functional (psychiatric), the concordance rate increased to 79%
> • the consultee's service; the results were broadly grouped into medical services (63%) and surgical services (11%)
> • the number of days of hospitalization; concordant cases were hospitalized fewer days at the time of the consult, spent fewer days in hospital after the consult, and had shorter overall admissions

In the 50% of cases that were NC, two-thirds made no mention of the diagnosis at all, while the other one-third contained inaccurate representations. Froese (1979) reported similar findings.

The sample of cases used in Callies (1980) was combined with those from another period of evaluation and published by Popkin (1983). The combination of cases was examined and yielded an overall concordance of 52%. A more detailed analysis of consulting services revealed the following rates of concordance:

- Neurosurgery   59%
- Other   58%
- General Medicine 56%
- Neurology   54%
- Gynecology   29%
- General Surgery   21%

The variables found to be significant in Callies (1980) were confirmed in this expanded sample.

In this study, diagnostic representation had the lowest concordance rate (52%) vs. 56% for diagnostic action and 69% for psychotropic drug recommendations.

In Popkin (1982), an assessment was made in randomly chosen cases as to whether the implemented diagnostic actions:

- clarified or changed the conceptualization of the case by the consultee (23%)
- made a contribution to ruling out a possible diagnosis or confirming an established or suspected one (73%)
- were represented in the discharge summary (23%)

Summary

Since diagnosis is a pivotal factor in outlining a treatment plan, it is surprising that representation on discharge summaries rated the lowest level of concordance. With omissions occurring twice as often as inaccurate descriptions, psychiatric diagnoses are often not seen as relevant information. This can also reflect a lack of interest towards, or comprehension of, psychiatric nosology — particularly on surgical services. Tests recommended by consultants that led to a reconceptualization of a case were even less likely to receive mention. With longer admissions, the amount of information summarized on discharge reports may preclude mention of a psychiatric consultation. The low level of diagnostic representation highlights the need for a thorough examination of patients' charts for previous psychiatric consultations.

References for Diagnostic Representation

A.L. Callies, M.L. Popkin, T.B. Mackenzie & J. Mitchell
Consultees' Representation of Consultants' Psychiatric Diagnoses
American Journal of Psychiatry 137(10): p. 1250 — 1253, 1980

A.P. Froese
Is The Psychiatrist's Opinion Heard?
Internat. Journal of Psychiatry in Medicine 8: p. 295 — 301, 1977-78

M.L. Popkin, T.B. Mackenzie, A.L. Callies & R.C.W. Hall
Yield of Psychiatric Consultants' Recommendations for Diagnostic Action
Archives of General Psychiatry 39: p. 843 — 845, 1982

M.L. Popkin, T.B. Mackenzie, A.L. Callies & R.C.W. Hall
Consultation-Liaison Outcome Evaluation System
Archives of General Psychiatry 40: p. 215 — 219, 1983

Sigmundoscopy — The Bases

◆ Psychiatry vs. Cardiology Consult Outcomes

Mackenzie (1981), in a diversification move that would have made a burger chain proud, applied CLOES methodology to assess concordance rates in a sample of cardiology consults.

Popkin (1981), compared the results from the above study to an equal number of psychiatric consults matched for hospital setting and time period. Frequency and concordance rates for medication and diagnostic action recommendations were compared.

The results were as follows for medication recommendations:
- **cardiac consults**   frequency 49%   concordance 82%
- **psych. consults**   frequency 45%   concordance 69%

While the difference in concordance rates was statistically significant, the difference in frequency was not.

The results for diagnostic action recommendations were:
- **cardiac consults**   frequency 38%   concordance 73%
- **psych. consults**   frequency 29%   concordance 56%

There was a significant difference for both the rates of diagnostic recommendations and concordance between these groups.

Popkin went on to elucidate the variables that were significant in determining the concordance for each type of recommendation and each service. The findings in this study did not vary from the positive findings outlined in the sections for medication recommendations and diagnostic actions for psychiatric consults.

The difference in concordance for medication recommendations was not found to be related to the identity of the consulting service. The factors relevant to concordance with cardiology consults had some overlap with those from psychiatry. When the type of drug recommendation was a "non-start" action (adjust, continue or stop) and multiple recommendations were made, concordance was higher for both services. The class of cardiac drug was a significant factor, which was not found in Popkin's results (though this was found to be an important factor in other studies).

Implementing the Treatment Plan

The factors that statistically increased concordance with diagnostic actions for cardiology consults were the presence of follow-up visits and the identity of the consult service. These factors were not the same in the psychiatry sample. The specific diagnostic action was unrelated to concordance in either group.

Summary
This study found overall that concordance was higher for cardiology consultations. Different sets of variables were important in determining the level of implementation between services.

References for Comparing Consult Outcomes
T.B. Mackenzie, M.L. Popkin, A.L. Callies et al
The Effectiveness of Cardiology Consultation
Chest 79: p. 16 — 22, 1981

M.L. Popkin, T.B. Mackenzie, A.L. Callies & J.N. Cohn
An Interdisciplinary Comparison of Consultation Outcomes
Archives of General Psychiatry 38: p. 821 — 825, 1981

◆ The Psychiatrist as Consultee

Hall (1980) found that almost half of a series of one hundred psychiatric patients from lower socioeconomic classes had coexisting physical problems that either caused or affected their psychiatric symptoms sufficiently that admission was necessary. An additional one-third of these patients suffered from medical illnesses severe enough to require medical treatment.

Mackenzie (1983) investigated the outcome of medical-surgical consults on a psychiatric inpatient unit. This article was a more detailed study of referral outcomes than was provided in an earlier article by Bernstein (1980), who reported that 25% of their series of psychiatric patients received medical-surgical consults.

Mackenzie found that 38% of the patients in his series received at least one consultation during their inpatient stay. The most common services involved were:

- Neurology   23%
- Gynecology   9%
- Endocrinology 9%

Additionally, three-quarters of all cardiology, endocrinology and neurology consults were requested within the first two weeks of admission. Recommendation rates were as follows:

- medication   27%
- diagnostic action 46%

All of the consultations contained a diagnostic impression. The concordance rates were as follows:

- medication recommendations   79%
- diagnostic action recommendations 75%
- diagnostic representation   61%

A summary of the Popkin and Mackenzie articles looking at concordance rates of psychiatric consults, medical-surgical consults to psychiatric units, and cardiology consults is as follows:

Frequency of Recommendations

	Consultant Psychiatrist^	Consultee Psychiatrist	Consultant Cardiologist^
Drug	45%	27%	49%
Diagnostic Action	29%	46%	38%

Concordance

	Consultant Psychiatrist[+]	Consultee Psychiatrist	Consultant Cardiologist^
Drug	63%	79%	82%
Diagnostic Action	53%	75%	73%
Diagnostic Representation	43%	61%	—

^ results from Popkin (1981)
+ results from Popkin (1983) using unadjusted rates

References for Psychiatrists as Consultees

R.A. Bernstein & D. Dreyfuss
Medical & Surgical Consultations to a General Hospital Psychiatry Unit
General Hospital Psychiatry 2: p. 267 — 270, 1980

R.C.W. Hall, E.R. Gardner, S.K. Stickney, A.F. LeCann & M.K. Popkin
Physical Illness Manifesting as Psychiatric Disease
Archives of General Psychiatry 37: p. 989 — 995, 1980

T.B. Mackenzie, M.L. Popkin, A.L. Callies & J. Kroll
Consultation Outcomes: The Psychiatrist as Consultee
Archives of General Psychiatry 40: p. 1211 — 1214, 1983

M.L. Popkin, T.B. Mackenzie, A.L. Callies & J.N. Cohn
An Interdisciplinary Comparison of Consultation Outcomes
Archives of General Psychiatry 38: p. 821— 825, 1981

M.L. Popkin, T.B. Mackenzie & A.L. Callies
Consultation-Liaison Outcome Evaluation System
Archives of General Psychiatry 40: p. 215 — 219, 1983

Other Positive Findings Regarding Concordance

"Positive findings" from other articles are listed in this section. By this, it is meant that the findings from studies having a significant effect on concordance are listed here. In many instances in the C-L literature, an article with certain findings can be negated by the findings of another. For example, where Popkin (1979) found that medication recommendations made in the first half of the admission had a higher concordance rate, Lanting (1984) found no such association. For this reason, the positive factors that had a bearing on concordance in at least one study are summarized to give a list of variables that *may* be important when considering concordance with your recommendations.

Lanting (1984) found that concordance for diagnostic action and representation was related to:

- the reason for referral, with the highest levels of concordance being found when the consults involved substance abuse or investigating a possible psychogenic cause for physical problems
- the type of referring service, with a rate of 60% for general medicine and 33% for general surgery
- the diagnosis of a somatoform mental disorder

Huyse (1992) determined the following factors were associated with increased concordance:

- the greater the number of recommendations
- a consultation performed earlier during the admission
- the higher the seniority/rank of the consultant

Huyse (1990) found the highest implementation rates for:

- determining the timing of discharge (96%)
- transfering care to another facility (95%)
- using restraints (89%)
- requesting other consultations (86%)
- arranging outpatient care (86%)
- increasing physical treatments (84%)

Implementing the Treatment Plan

The lowest concordance rates in this study were for the following interventions:

- re-orienting cognitively impaired patients (21%)
- obtaining information from the family physician (40%)
- providing objects to help re-orient patients (e.g. clock, newspapers, calendar) (48%)
- obtaining information from the patient's family (52%)

Wise (1987) found that adjustment disorders and dysthymic disorders were the most likely to be omitted from discharge summaries. Neurosurgery and oncology referring sources were the most likely to omit psychiatric discharge diagnoses.

Wise (1987) also noted that 63% of patients' primary psychiatric diagnoses were missing from the admission note. Organic mental disorders, dementia and substance abuse were the most likely conditions to be omitted.

References for Concordance Studies
F.J. Huyse, J.J. Strain & J.S. Hammer
Interventions in Consultation-Liaison Psychiatry
General Hospital Psychiatry 12: p. 221 — 231, 1990

F.J. Huyse, J.S. Lyons & J.J. Strain
Evaluating Psychiatric Consultations in the General Hospital
General Hospital Psychiatry 14: p. 363 — 369, 1992

R.H.H. Lanting & M.W. Hengeveld
Outcome of Psychiatric Consultation in a Dutch University Hospital
Psychosomatics 25(8): p. 619 — 625, 1984

M.L. Popkin, T.B. Mackenzie, R.C.W. Hall & J.G. Garrard
Physicians' Concordance With Consultants' Recommendations For Psychotropic Medication
Archives of General Psychiatry 36: p. 386 — 389, 1979

T.N. Wise, L.S. Mann, R. Silverstein & J. Steg
CLOES: Resident or Private Attending Physicians' Concordance With Consultants' Recommendations
Comprehensive Psychiatry 28(5): p. 430 — 436, 1987

A Synthesis of Concordance Findings

As mentioned previously, it is difficult to define a coherent set of features that predict concordance for recommendation in an individual consult. For this reason, the preceding sections have listed factors associated with positive outcome in various studies and not a critical review of the merits of each study.

A generalizable finding from the C-L literature is that **process variables** are the most significant in determining concordance. For example, the timing of the consult during the admission, identity of the referring service and age of the patient seem to have more to do with the implementation of recommendations than the patient's medical problem, the patient's psychiatric diagnosis (other than OMD) or the seniority/status of the consultant.

Local factors also play a large part in concordance. For example, Huyse (1992) was the only psychiatric consultant involved in his study, and he reported a special arrangement with the otolaryngology department (giving an overrepresentation of such patients). These "local factors" affect the study results to an extent that large differences in concordance are seen in the literature. For this reason, it is imperative to have an awareness of which of the factors listed (or not listed) are relevant to your service.

A second consistent principle from outcome studies is that consultees are more interested in recommendations involving patient management than in diagnostic evaluation. Huyse (1990) found the highest concordance for discharge recommendations, and other studies support the finding that these suggestions are almost always carried out.

While Popkin (1980) stated that a psychiatry consult is largely viewed as a nonmedical intervention, it also appears that referring sources prematurely end the medical investigation of patients with psychiatric symptoms. When OMD was diagnosed, concordance rose appreciably, in keeping with the medical model approach to understanding illness.

Implementing the Treatment Plan

Concordance is higher with recommendations for single events with direct, tangible results and that involve activities that are usually performed by consultees. For example, psychological management of patients on the ward and obtaining psychosocial information are less likely to be implemented.

Services having a greater overlap with psychiatry are more likely to implement recommendations and record discharge diagnoses. This has a particular relevance to surgical services, who consistently rated the lowest in these areas.

The timing of consult requests is an important factor, but has two aspects. Early requests may indicate:

- a greater appreciation for psychosocial issues
- that the medical management is not yet firmly established and the consultee is more open to your input

Early requests also have the practical advantage that there is a longer time period in which recommendations can be implemented. On the other hand, consult recommendations involving patients with longer-term hospital stays or complex situations are also associated with higher levels of implementation. While there is some debate, making multiple recommendations appears to increase concordance, possibly because this indicates your active involvement in the patient's care.

References for Concordance

F.J. Huyse, J.J. Strain & J.S. Hammer
Interventions in Consultation-Liaison Psychiatry
General Hospital Psychiatry 12: p. 221 — 231, 1990

F.J. Huyse, J.S. Lyons & J.J. Strain
Evaluating Psychiatric Consultations in the General Hospital
General Hospital Psychiatry 14: p. 363 — 369, 1992

M.L. Popkin, T.B. Mackenzie & A. L. Callies
Consultees' Concordance With Consultants' Recommendations For Diagnostic Action
Journal of Nervous and Mental Disorders 168(1): p. 9 — 12, 1980

Why Would Consultees Not Implement Recommendations?

As outlined in Chapter Three, the biases that influence requests for psychiatric consultation continue to make an impact on the implementation of recommendations. Some of these factors apply to consults in general, while others apply to psychiatric consults specifically.

◆ **Factors that Apply to Consults in General**

• unfortunately, some consultants reinforce their expert status by making recommendations that are poorly conceived, not essential, and may not even be helpful

• recommendations may be poorly explained or deemed not pertinent to the patient's care; additionally, consultees may lack the skills to perform certain actions (e.g. a thorough mental status exam)

• the higher costs involved in implementing tests are a factor, though Popkin (1981) found that more expensive procedures had a higher likelihood of implementation

• representation may be deficient because physicians are taught to be conservative with their diagnoses and to search for a single condition which explains all of a patient's symptoms; in cases of serious illness, it may seem sufficient to record that the patient survived and list only the factors directly related to the physical aspects of recovery

Lee (1983), found complete disagreement between consultant and consultee regarding the reason for referral (principal clinical issue) in 14% of cases. In these situations, there was significantly less usefulness attributed to the consult in assisting with diagnosis or management. Although this study did not monitor concordance, it is likely that the implementation of recommendations was lower when the consult wasn't perceived as being helpful. Interestingly, house officers rated an average of 7% of the consults they requested as being either "superfluous" or "for educational value only" even when there was agreement on the reason for consultation.

Implementing the Treatment Plan

◆ Factors Specific to Psychiatric Consultations
- of all the medical specialties, psychiatry has the greatest range of reasons for which consultation is requested; if the referring source is seeking help with patient management (e.g. acting as a buffer or intermediary in dealing with difficult aspects or facilitating transfer or discharge), recommendations for diagnostic action may be seen as being beyond the scope of the consultation

- the request for a psychiatric consult may be a signal to indicate the end of the patient's organic investigation

- if referring sources have made an oversight, it may be less palatable to have a psychiatric service discover this than another physical medicine specialty

- psychiatry may not be viewed as being scientific enough, or that a psychiatric diagnosis is nothing more than a subjective opinion; the diagnostic rationale and nosology are less likely to be understood by non-psychiatric physicians who may be uncomfortable with merely echoing the impression from the consult note

- one of the most enduring pieces of information physicians retain about psychiatric medications is that they can cause a diverse number of side effects; consultees may be reluctant to start psychotropic medications for fear that this could interfere with existing medical treatments or cause complications that will prolong the patient's stay (e.g. neuroleptic malignant syndrome)

- consultees may be seeking affirmation that the patient presents a challenging case and that they require reassurance that they're doing a thorough job; in a related instance, occasionally a **negative consult** is sought, in which the referring source seeks assurances that nothing has been missed or that nothing more can be done for the patient

- local or process aspects may apply, resulting in an arbitrary degree of concordance; while these factors are largely beyond the consultees' control, it is still important to be aware of them, and to periodically let referring sources know that you are monitoring the effectiveness of your recommendations

Sigmundoscopy — The Bases

◆ *Is there an optimum level of concordance?*
In Mackenzie (1983), psychiatrists didn't completely implement management suggestions when requesting consults. Rather, concordance was found to be 79% for drug recommendations and 75% for diagnostic actions. Popkin (1981) found that cardiologists enjoyed concordance rates of 82% for treatment recommendations and 73% for diagnostic actions. These rates are an important guide because there is less of a disparity in the expertise in physical medicine between consultant and consultee in these cases.

Lee (1983) studied house officers' perceptions of the value of a consultation for the purpose of diagnosis and management. He found that 77% were rated as either crucial, contributory or confirmatory for diagnosis and 82% for management. In cases where there is agreement on these matters, the referring team is much more likely to implement suggestions. Pooling these findings, it appears that concordance rates of between 75% to 85% are what our colleagues are achieving.

A concordance rate of 100% is not obtainable in hospitals where recommendations must be approved before they can be implemented. For clinical, legal and ethical reasons, primary physicians retain control of their patients' management and do not simply turn it over to the various consultants whom they ask for advice. Discretion in implementing suggestions indicates that consultees critically review the care they provide for their patients, and that consults are one aspect of this process.

Legal aspects pertaining to the degree of consultee's concordance are discussed in the next chapter.

Summary
Popkin (1980) noted that the implementation rates were not related to the type of diagnostic action recommended. Because there was as much resistance to recommendations for psychological testing as there was to other investigations, he felt the disinterest was not based on psychiatrists' competence in requesting tests. Rather, he stated that "*the phenomenon seems to be a disincli-*

nation engendered by the very act of seeking a psychiatric consultation."

The studies discussed in this chapter reveal significantly higher concordance rates for cardiology consults. The degree of concordance shown by psychiatrists when requesting consults was very close to that obtained by the cardiologists. Based on the findings of the studies presented in this chapter, it appears that psychiatric C-L services face unique difficulties regarding concordance. The biases that exist against even requesting consults continue to exert an influence that limits the implementation of recommendations and ultimately the usefulness of psychiatric interventions.

References for Nonconcordance
T. Lee, E.M. Pappius & L. Goldman
Impact of Inter-Physician Communication on the Effectiveness of Medical Consultations
The American Journal of Medicine 74: p. 106 — 112, 1983

T.B. Mackenzie, M.L. Popkin, A.L. Callies & J. Kroll
Consultation Outcomes: The Psychiatrist As Consultee
Archives of General Psychiatry 40: p. 1211— 1214, 1983

M.L. Popkin, T.B. Mackenzie, & A.L. Callies
Consultees' Concordance With Consultants' Recommendations For Diagnostic Action
Journal of Nervous and Mental Disorders 168(1): p. 9 — 12, 1980

M.L. Popkin, T.B. Mackenzie & A.L. Callies
Improving the Effectiveness of Psychiatric Consultation
Psychosomatics 22(7): p. 559 — 563, 1981

M.L. Popkin, T.B. Mackenzie, A.L. Callies & J.N. Cohn
An Interdisciplinary Comparison of Consultation Outcomes
Archives of General Psychiatry 38: p. 821 — 825, 1981

Sigmundoscopy — The Bases

Strategies to Improve Concordance

Studies have consistently found that process and local variables are more important than clinical variables in determining concordance. Consultants need to be aware of interventions that will increase concordance by altering the consultation process.

◆ **Recommendations**
- where multiple recommendations are made, list the most important one(s) first
- Wise (1987) found that the number of recommendations averaged between 1—3 for the consult note and initial note and 1—2 on follow-up visits
- use a clearly demarcated section of your consult report to list recommendations
- be specific and brief
- be decisive; avoid conditional suggestions
- keep concordance rates in mind; explain your rationale for recommendations less likely to be implemented

◆ **Follow-up Visits**
- Sensky (1986) reported that for two-thirds of consult patients, only two visits were made
- making follow-up visits and leaving progress notes has been correlated with increasing concordance (use these visits to remind referring sources about your suggestions)
- following patients conveys your interest and allows you to evaluate the effectiveness of your interventions
- if primary physicians are aware you are monitoring concordance, it may increase

◆ **Assign Responsibility**
- most interventions are best made by specific people
- contract with consultees regarding who will carry out your recommendations (you, physician, nurse, etc.)
- the more the intervention departs from the person's usual activities, the less likely it is to be implemented
- you may need to teach others (or arrange for instruction) the first time a task is performed

Implementing the Treatment Plan

◆ Structure Your Approach
- use reminders
- tailor the treatment to fit the referring source
- introduce components sequentially where possible
- monitor the results personally
- provide positive feedback to the consultees

◆ Ask About Nonconcordance
- Popkin allowed 96 hours for implementation; the first and last 24 hours of an admission are time periods where compliance is likely to be low
- ask consultees about their rationale for not implementing your recommendations — it is the only way you will discover the local and process variables operating with that referring source at your hospital
- because a degree of nonconcordance is expected, approach the problem as an intellectual curiosity, not as a comment on your ability or about you personally
- advocate for your recommendations; Guggenheim (1978) said *"the inexperienced consultant places little emphasis on selling suggestions to the consultee and does not try to overcome the mild suspicion with which consultees often regard consultations of all specialties."*

References for Improving Concordance

F. Guggenheim
A Marketplace Model of Consultation Psychiatry
American Journal of Psychiatry 135(11): p. 1380 — 1383, 1978

R.B. Haynes, D.W. Taylor & D.L. Sackett
Compliance in Health Care
Johns Hopkins University Press, Baltimore, 1979

T. Sensky
The General Hospital Psychiatrist: Too Many Tasks And Too Few Roles?
British Journal of Psychiatry 148: p. 151 — 158, 1986

T.N. Wise, L.S. Mann, R. Silverstein & J. Steg
CLOES: Resident or Private Attending Physicians' Concordance With Consultants' Recommendations
Comprehensive Psychiatry 28(5): p. 430 — 436, 1987

◆ Ten Commandments (C-L Version)

- determine the question
- establish urgency
- look for yourself
- be as brief as appropriate
- be specific
- provide contingency plans
- honor thy turf (or thou shalt not covet thy neighbor's patient)
- teach. . . with tact
- talk is cheap. . . and effective
- follow-up

L. Goldman, T. Lee & P. Rudd
Ten Commandments For Effective Consultations
Archives of Internal Medicine 143: p. 1753 — 1755, 1983
© American Medical Association, Used with permission

◆ Ten More Commandments

- thou shalt love thy fellow physician as thyself
- thou shalt not procrastinate
- thou shalt not obfuscate
- thou shalt be concrete
- thou shalt honor thy patient's spouse, children, and parents
- thou shalt not hibernate
- thou shalt persevere
- thou shalt not preach
- thou shalt not steal thy fellow physician's patients
- thou shalt not shirk thy duty to thy hospital medical staff or thy local medical society

The last point is especially significant. The author points out that the lack of a psychiatric presence contributes to *"the aloofness and distance that has plagued our specialty."* Increased visibility helps others keep us in mind for future consult requests.

R.O. Pasnau
Ten Commandments of Medical Etiquette for Psychiatrists
Psychosomatics 26(2): p. 128 — 132, 1985
© American Psychiatric Press, Inc., Used with permission

Other References Dealing with Concordance

F.J. Huyse, J.J. Strain & J.S. Hammer
Interventions in Consultation-Liaison Psychiatry, Part I: Patterns of Recommendations
General Hospital Psychiatry 12: 213 — 220, 1990

T.B. Karasu, R. Plutchik, H. Conte, B. Siegel et al
What Do Physicians Want From A Psychiatric Consultation Service?
Comprehensive Psychiatry 18: p. 73 — 81, 1977

A.J. Krakowski
Psychiatric Consultation in the General Hospital: An Exploration of Resistances
Diseases of the Nervous System 36: p. 242 — 244, 1975

T.B. Mackenzie, M.K. Popkin & A.L. Callies
CLOES, Part I: Teaching Applications
Journal of Nervous and Mental Disorders 169(10): p. 648 — 653, 1981

K.R. Özbayrak
Concordance: Sequencing of Psychiatric Recommendations (letter)
Psychosomatics 35(2): p. 171 — 172, 1994

T.L. Thompson II, T.N. Wise & A.B. Kelley et al
Improving Psychiatric Consultation to Non-Psychiatric Physicians
Psychosomatics 31: p. 80 — 84, 1990

S.J. Schleifer, S. Bhardwaj, A. Lebovits et al
Predictors of Physician Nonadherence to Chemotherapy Regimens
Cancer 67: p. 945 — 951, 1991

C. van Dyke, D. Rice, P. Pallett & H. Leigh
Psychiatric Consultation: Compliance and Level of Satisfaction With Recommendations
Psychother. Psychosom. 33: p. 14 — 24, 1980

Sigmundoscopy — The Bases

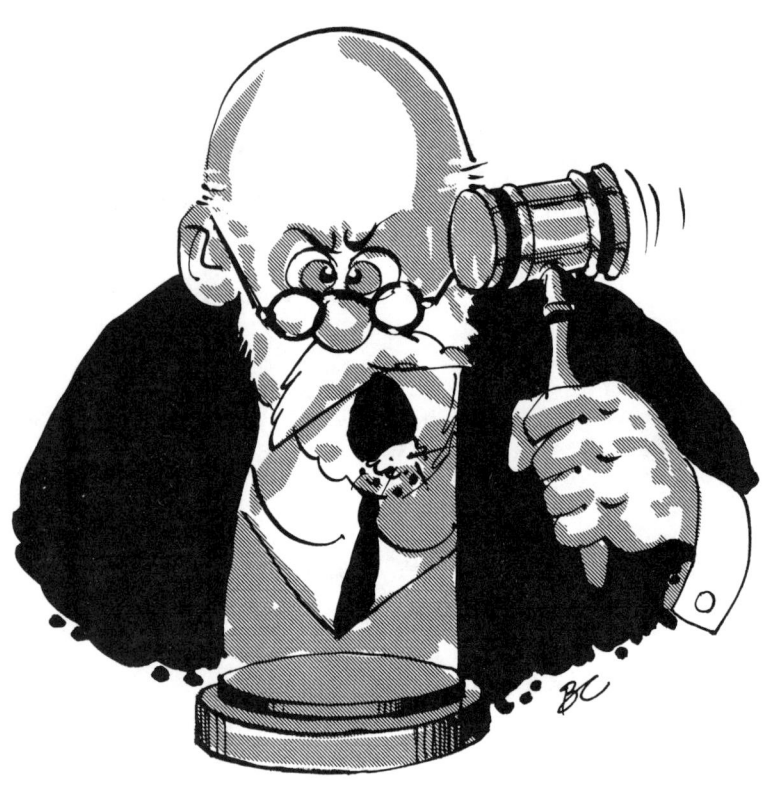

Legal & Ethical Aspects

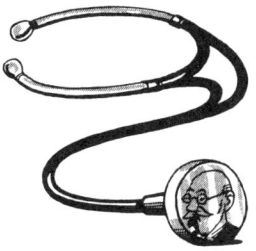

6/ Legal & Ethical Aspects

The medicolegal liability incurred by C-L activities merits further consideration. C-L psychiatrists practice under conditions which are suboptimal, particularly when performing assessments on busy wards and lobbying to have treatment recommendations implemented. Psychiatric involvement with most medical/surgical patients involves what is practical instead of ideal, and must balance the needs of each party involved in the consult process.

For the most part, psychiatrists encounter fewer malpractice lawsuits than most other specialists (as can be gauged by insurance fees). The reasons for this are varied:

- some patients may be reluctant to terminate their relationship with a psychiatrist by launching a lawsuit
- psychiatrists do not perform invasive procedures and do not independently treat physically ill patients
- treatments generally take place over days to weeks to months, leaving ample opportunity for monitoring and intervention
- in some cases, it is debatable how much "loss" occurs or to what extent a patient's long-term functioning will be impaired by psychiatric treatments

It may seem that C-L psychiatrists, who work in less than ideal conditions with physically ill patients, incur a greater medicolegal risk. However, Garrick (1994) indicates that at the time he wrote his article, there were no published legal cases where psychiatrists were held liable for negligent consultations, though he cautions that many claims are settled out of court.

Sigmundoscopy — The Bases

There are a multitude of medicolegal factors in C-L work, many of which have been addressed in the chapters on the consultation process, documentation and implementation of recommendations. The responsibility assumed by psychiatrists varies on a case-by-case basis because each consultation involves a unique set of circumstances. For this reason, it is not possible to provide an all-inclusive set of guidelines addressing medicolegal risks.

The following factors are relevant in determining risk and culpability in all C-L activities:

◆ **Establishing a Doctor-Patient Relationship (DPR)**
Liaison activities such as general seminar series, without focus on actual patients, would not constitute a DPR. Liaison activities geared towards particular patients, even if the psychiatrist has not yet seen the person, increases liability. For example **curbside consultations** involve questions about patients in which the consultant does not have the opportunity to conduct an interview or review the chart. This situation can present medicolegal risks for the consultant and should be dealt with in one of two ways: either advising that a formal consultation be requested, or clearly establishing that your recommendations are of a general nature and not intended for a specific patient.

Clearly the act of performing a consultation establishes a DPR. Irwin (1985) indicates that a DPR is established when a bill is submitted for services rendered (curbside consultations are rarely billed). However, responsibility to the patient may be considered to begin when a consult is requested, not when the patient is first seen (hence the need for timely responses).

◆ **Degree of Responsibility**
A greater degree of involvement in a patient's care brings about a greater liability. For example, a consult requested to recommend a dosage for a medication that a patient is already taking (but has forgotten) involves less medicolegal responsibility than taking over the care of that patient and by transferring her to the psychiatry unit. For this reason, it is crucial to understand what level of in-

Legal & Ethical Aspects

volvement is being requested by the referring source. Liability is reduced in situations involving more precise consult requests and less contact with patients.

◆ *Special Expertise*

C-L psychiatrists are assumed to have knowledge and abilities beyond that of the physicians requesting the consult. For this reason, it is expected that all physicians be aware of their limitations and request assistance for matters beyond their professional knowledge. It is also a good practice to inform patients of this situation and advise them that the assistance of others is necessary. Further, the person conducting the consult is expected to provide services at a level of skill comparable to others who have the same training. For example, a hospital that uses general psychiatrists on a rotating basis for consultation duties would be held to a lower standard than one in a university teaching center with an established C-L service. Liability also increases if the psychiatrist with the highest degree of skill is not informed of a situation requiring his or her attention.

◆ *Duty to the Patient*

C-L psychiatrists have an obligation to explain to patients the diagnoses that are made and treatments that are instituted. Consultees do not have the expertise to advise patients about psychiatric illnesses. Even though consultees usually retain the ultimate authority for instituting treatment, they do not often explain the risks and benefits to patients in sufficient detail to obtain **informed consent**. It is prudent to make it clear who will be obtaining consent from the patient (a task which is usually delegated to the person who is most knowledgeable in the area).

Because referring sources will often have not told patients about the consult, or even the need for one, it is helpful to explain that the role of a consultant is to assist the primary physician.

Confidentiality is also a duty to patients (discussed previously). By reiterating the role of a consultant, patients gain a clearer idea about who has access to the information they share with you.

Sigmundoscopy — The Bases

◆ Duty to the Consultee

Due to the lack of guidance from the medicolegal literature, it is at times unclear towards whom consult activities are geared. While patients' best interests are clearly important, there are a number of obligations to keep in mind for referring sources:

- assuming responsibility for certain tasks because of the skills possessed by psychiatrists (e.g. ECT, psychotherapy)

- accepting the responsibility for recommendations which are implemented and following patients' progress (because consultees are jointly liable with consultants for damages)

- making consultees aware of situations in which patients' mental state or emotional reaction to their illness impairs the delivery of medical care (e.g. a patient wishing to sign out of hospital)

- informing the primary physician when his or her actions may result in harm to the patient (e.g. a deteriorating relationship with the patient that may result in suboptimal care)

- assessing patients' capacity to consent to treatment and assisting in the legal process for obtaining substitute consent (where necessary); advising consultees on the urgent treatment of involuntary or incapable patients (e.g. physical restraints)

- realizing the physician has asked for an opinion on a patient's management and not for the transfer of care; assisting the primary physician to integrate the advice from all sources to deliver the most appropriate treatment

- not withstanding the above, it is important to monitor whether or not your recommendations have been implemented

- investigating nonconcordance to make certain that consultees are making informed decisions (instead of being unfamiliar with or minimizing psychiatric problems), and imparting to consultees that they risk liability when they don't have valid reasons for not following your advice

- if patients declined consultations, all parties involved should be made aware of the risks involved in not participating

Legal & Ethical Aspects

◆ Duty to Hospital & Society
Patients need to be protected when, because of a mental illness, they pose a risk to themselves, others, or are unable to care for themselves outside of a structured setting. These risks are not always apparent to consultees. When information is obtained that indicates the patient is not capable of performing certain tasks (i.e. driving a car, flying an airplane), the proper authorities need to be notified. Similarly, when there is evidence (or in some areas, just the suspicion) of child or elder abuse, this too must be reported.

◆ Duty to Trainees
Supervisors are legally responsible for the actions of their trainees, even if the patient wasn't seen directly. This is called the principle of **respondeat superior**.

◆ Documentation
Medical records are legal documents that serve a number of purposes beyond being a record of the care provided. Charts are the only records accepted in court. As such, they are a medicolegal benefit if they contain the following:

- detailed descriptions of the signs and symptoms used to delineate psychiatric illness and pathological biological and psychosocial processes, and a mental status examination
- difficulties encountered when assessing patients
- a cataloging of risks and benefits, and the reasoning behind taking a course of action
- a close correlation between actions and documentation

The **Joint Commission on Accreditation of Hospital Standards in the Accreditation Manual for Hospitals** sets standards for documentation that are widely used and updated yearly.

◆ Selection of Consultants
Physicians are expected to obtain assistance from appropriate professionals, which highlights the need for C-L teams with a complement of professionals from a variety of disciplines who can handle all clinical situations, and formulate and implement a comprehensive biopsychosocial treatment plan.

Ethical Aspects

Confidentiality is the professional obligation to not disclose information shared by patients, and is particularly important to psychiatrists whose work is dependent on patients' trust. Confidentiality is not absolute, particularly in consultations where the assessment provides information for referring sources. Breeches of confidentiality are justified when there are deemed to be risks to third parties, both identifiable and unidentifiable. In some cases, there are legal requirements for psychiatrists to reveal information. In other cases, the management of confidentiality is *"much more a matter of professional ethics."* (Joseph, 1993)

Kaplan & Sadock (1998) identify two main theories which guide the ethical treatment of patients in psychiatry:

- **Utilitarian Theory** — the main goal in decision making is to produce the greatest degree of happiness for the largest number of people; this theory also encompasses the concept of **paternalism**, in which physicians have a duty of beneficence towards their patients, as do parents for their children

- **Autonomy Theory** — patients are presumed to have the ability to make decisions and are given legal rights to do so; while this theory takes into account the potential for patients' decisions being in their best interests, it does not require that people are forced to achieve this goal if they wish otherwise

C-L psychiatrists are commonly faced with issues related to **informed consent**. This involves individuals making voluntary decisions, in an atmosphere free of coercion and duress, about their care, having been provided with relevant information regarding their diagnosis and prognosis, the risks and benefits of proposed treatments, and of alternative choices. The following factors are taken into account when evaluating patients' competency to make treatment decisions (Appelbaum, 1987):

- communication of a choice
- ability to understand the information disclosed about a proposed treatment
- ability to appreciate the implications of alternative choices
- ability to make a reasonable treatment decision

Legal References

T.R. Garrick & R. Weinstock
Liability of Psychiatric Consultants
Psychosomatics 35(5): p. 474 — 484, 1994

J.R. Irwin
Legal Implications of Intraoperative Consultation
Urology Clinics of North America 12: p. 557 — 570, 1985

Joint Commission of Accreditation of Hospitals
Joint Commission of Accreditation of Health Care Organizations: Accreditation Manual for Hospitals
Chicago, 1989

Ethics References

P.S. Appelbaum, C.W. Lidz & A. Meisel
Informed Consent: Legal Theory and Clinical Practice
Oxford University Press, New York, 1987

American Psychiatric Association
The Principles of Medical Ethics: With Annotations Especially Applicable to Psychiatry
American Psychiatric Press, Inc., Washington D.C., 1993

S.A. Green
The Ethical Limits of Confidentiality in the Therapeutic Relationship
General Hospital Psychiatry 17: p. 80 — 84, 1995

D. Joseph & J. Onek
Confidentiality in Psychiatry, in
Psychiatric Ethics, Second Edition
S. Bloch & P. Chodoff, Editors
Oxford University Press, Oxford, England, 1993

H.I. Kaplan & B.J. Sadock, Editors
Synopsis of Psychiatry, Eighth Edition
Williams & Wilkins, Baltimore, 1998

D. Robinson & C. Garratt
Ethics for Beginners
Icon Book, Cambridge, England, 1996

The Consultation Process

The Referral

Obtain the following information at the time the consultation is requested:

"I'M SURE"

Identifying Factors
Medical Problem(s)

Source of Referral
Urgency
Reason for Referral
Expectations of the Consultee

Preparing for the Consult

Consider the four entities involved in the consultation:
- Patient
- Consultee
- Reason for Referral
- C-L Service

Before seeing the patient:
- Refresh your knowledge of the medical/surgical illness
- Contact the ward
- Read the chart

Interviewing the Patient

The C-L Interview:
- Explain the purpose and limitations of the interview
- Spend time developing rapport by discussing the physical illness
- Try to find a private area to conduct the interview
- Your priority is to answer the consultation question
- Be flexible in your interview style

The Consultation Process

The Consult Note

- Title, date, time, location
- Your name, rank and phone #
- Sources of information

- Relevant personal information about the patient and a synopsis of the medical/surgical problem
- Restate (or state) the purpose for the consultation and the expectations of the consultee

- A pertinent history incorporating biopsychosocial factors
- Eliciting symptoms and distillation of a diagnostic impression
- A personal history including reactions to stress and illness, substance use, legal problems, etc.

- Screening questions to search for comorbid conditions
- List significant negatives
- Perform a MSE on all patients

- Provide an impression, summary or formulation
- List the impediments in obtaining information (if any)
- Sign your note

Implementing Recommendations

- Develop a biopsychosocial management plan involving investigations, short and longer term treatments

- Clearly indicate who should be making the above interventions

- Speak to consultees directly about urgent concerns

- Monitor concordance

From **Sigmundocopy, The Bases** by David J. Robinson M.D., © Rapid Psychler Press

Sigmundoscopy — The Bases

Index

Academy of Psychosomatic Medicine (APM)   4, 34, 38, 42, 43, 64
Accreditation Council for Graduate Medical Education (ACGME)   33
American Association of Directors of Psychiatric Residency Training (AADPRT)   34
American Board of Medical Specialties (ABMS)   44, 45
American Board of Psychiatry & Neurology (ABPN)   44
American Hospital Association (AHA)   4
American Medical Association (AMA)   27, 131
American Neurologic Association (ANA)   27
American Psychiatric Association (APA)   4, 34, 42, 44
American Psychosomatic Society (APS)   13, 19, 43
Anna O   16
Association for Academic Psychiatry (AAP)   34
Autonomonic Nervous System   18 — 21
Autonomy Theory   176
Biopsychosocial
    approach   3, 31
    grid   119
    management plan   117 — 131
CLOES
    defined   147
Comorbidity   62 — 3, 70
Concordance
    defined   145
   146—153, 158—161, 164, 166 — 7
Confidentiality   173, 176
Consultation Psychiatry
    defined   8 — 9
    models   8 — 9

Consultations
    benefits   64, 67— 68
    cardiology   154 — 5
    clarity of requests   78 — 80
    commandments   168
    commodity model   104 — 5
    common requests   57
    conducting   75 — 107
    curbside   75, 172
    diagnoses seen   61
    documenting   131 — 141
    duties   173 — 5
    ethical aspects   176
    expectations   81
    implementation of recommendations   162 — 165
    interviewing patients   88 — 103
    legal aspects   171 — 5
    local variables   60, 162 — 5
    negative   163
    notification   88 — 9
    outcome evaluation   56
    overlooking   69
    preparation   83 — 7
    process   34, 178 — 9
    process variables   60, 162 — 165
    rates of   60
    recommendations   116 — 143
    reporting   109 — 143
    requested by psychiatrists   156 — 7
    resistance to   78
    sample notes   132 — 140
    use   57
    usefulness   56
Consultation-Liaison (C-L) Psychiatry
    abilities needed   5, 6, 31, 58
    bibliographies   35
    composition   39
    defined   3 — 4, 13, 60
    education   33 — 4, 45 — 6
    funding   38
    future   46
    history   26 — 30

Index

name change 7
outpatient 40 — 1
practice guidelines 42 — 3
practitioners 4
qualities needed 32
range of activities 5
research 36 — 7, 45
subspecialty status 44 — 5
teaching guidelines 33 — 5
Conversion Reaction 18, 23
Cost-Benefit Analysis 64
Cost-Effectiveness Analysis 65 — 8
Cost Offset Study 65
Doctor-Patient Relationship (DPR) 172
Epidemiology
consultations 61
psychiatric illnesses 59
Ethical Aspects 176
Factitious Disorder 23
Fight-Flight Reaction 18, 20
Health Care Financing Administration (HCFA) 131
Hypochondriasis 23
Hysteria 17
Informed Consent 173, 176
Interviewing Patients
initiating 90 — 1
outline 92 — 5
priorities 94
references 99
vignette 100 — 3
Investigations
biological 86, 117, 122 — 4
psychosocial 117, 125
Learning Theory 20
Liaison Psychiatry
defined 10 — 11, 60
Malingering 23
Medications 118 — 9, 126 — 9
Mental Status Examination (MSE) 31, 95, 97, 98, 110, 114
Mini-Mental State Exam (MMSE) 82, 114

Mnemonics
Consult Referral 76
Medical Differential Diagnosis 120
MSE 98
Organic Considerations 124
Treatment Modes 121
Multidisciplinary Theories 18, 21
National Institute of Mental Health (NIMH) 30, 66
Nonspecificity Theories 18, 20
Prevention
Primary 10
Secondary 9
Tertiary 9
Psychobiology 27, 28
Psychological Factors Affecting Medical Conditions (PFAMC) 24 — 5
Psychological Testing 125
Psychotherapy 56, 118, 119, 130
Psychopharmacology 86, 119, 126 — 9
Psychosomatic Medicine
conditions 21
current concepts 22 — 3
general 3, 13, 22
history 14 — 21
Referral Parameters 76 — 82
Regression 97
Reports (Consult)
goals 110 — 1
overview 109, 142
sections 112 — 5
Representation 146, 152 — 3
Royal College of Physicians & Surgeons of Canada (RCPSC) 33, 44
Secondary Gain 23
Social investigations 117, 125
treatments 118, 119, 130 — 1
Somatoform Disorders 23
Specificity Theories 18, 19
Splitting 96, 130
Transference 16
Treatment Plan Implementation 162 — 5
Utilitarian Theory 176

The Author

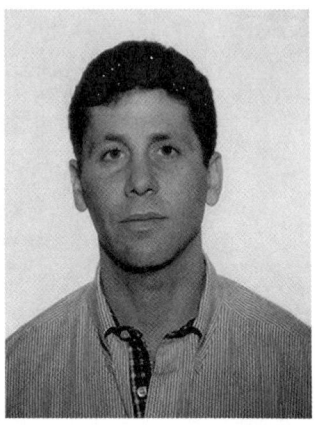

Dave Robinson is a psychiatrist practicing in London, Ontario, Canada. His particular interests are consultation-liaison psychiatry and both undergraduate and postgraduate education. A graduate of the University of Toronto Medical School, he completed a Residency in Family Practice before entering the Psychiatry Residency Program. He is a Lecturer in the Department of Psychiatry at the University of Western Ontario in London, Canada.

The Artist

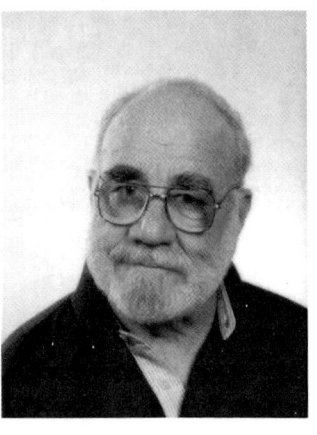

Brian Chapman is a resident of Oakville, Ontario, Canada. He was born in Sussex, England and moved to Canada in 1957. His first commercial work took place during W.W. II when he traded drawings for cigarettes while serving in the British Navy. Now retired, Brian was formerly a Creative Director at Mediacom. He continues to freelance and is versatile in a wide range of media. He is a master of the caricature, and his talents are constantly in demand. He doesn't smoke anymore. Brian is an avid swimmer and trumpeter. He performs regularly (playing the trumpet) in the Toronto area as a member of three bands. He is married to Fanny, a cook, bridge player and crossword puzzle solver extraordinaire.

Rapid Psychler Press was founded in 1994 with the aim of producing textbooks and resource materials that further the use of humor in mental health education. In addition to textbooks, Rapid Psychler specializes in producing CD-ROMs, slides and overheads for presentations.

Rapid Psychler Press